T0234823

Successful Accreditation in Echocardiography

Successful Accreditation in Echocardiography
A Self-Assessment Guide

**Sanjay M. Banypersad MBChB,
BMedSci (Hons), MRCP (UK)**
Cardiology SpR
The Heart Hospital
London
UK

Keith Pearce
Principal Cardiac Physiologist
Wythenshawe Hospital
Manchester
UK

Endorsed by the British Society
of Echocardiography

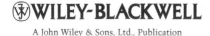

A John Wiley & Sons, Ltd., Publication

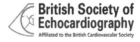

British Society of
Echocardiography
Affiliated to the British Cardiovascular Society

This edition first published 2012 © 2012 by John Wiley & Sons, Ltd.

Wiley-Blackwell is an imprint of John Wiley & Sons, formed by the merger of Wiley's global Scientific, Technical and Medical business with Blackwell Publishing.

Registered Office:
John Wiley & Sons, Ltd, The Atrium, Southern Gate, Chichester, West Sussex, PO19 8SQ, UK

Editorial Offices:
9600 Garsington Road, Oxford, OX4 2DQ, UK
111 River Street, Hoboken, NJ 07030-5774, USA

For details of our global editorial offices, for customer services and for information about how to apply for permission to reuse the copyright material in this book please see our website at www.wiley.com/wiley-blackwell

Library of Congress Cataloging-in-Publication Data

Banypersad, Sanjay M.
Successful accreditation in echocardiography : a self-assessment guide / Sanjay M. Banypersad, Keith Pearce.
    p. ; cm.
  Includes index.
  ISBN-13: 978-0-4706-5692-1 (pbk. : alk. paper)
  ISBN-10: 0-470-65692-1 (pbk. : alk. paper)
I. Pearce, Keith (Keith A.)   II. Title.
[DNLM: 1. Echocardiography–Examination Questions. WG 18.2]
  LC classification not assigned
  616.1'2307543076–dc23

                         2011029720

A catalogue record for this book is available from the British Library.

Wiley also publishes its books in a variety of electronic formats. Some content that appears in print may not be available in electronic books.

Set in 9.25/12pt Meridien by SPi Publisher Services, Pondicherry, India

1 2012

Contents

9 Video Questions

COMPANION WEBSITE

This book is accompanied by a companion website:

www.accreditationechocardiography.com

The website includes:

- 89 interactive Multiple-Choice Questions
- 193 Videoclips

Foreword

Echocardiography is a mainstay of cardiac diagnostics and remains by far the most commonly performed imaging examination in cardiology practice. The development of easily portable and hand held machines has enhanced its use in bedside diagnosis and emergency assessment while real time 3-D imaging, tissue Doppler and speckle tracking provide a sophisticated insight into myocardial structure and function. In tandem with the development of technology has come the recognition that echocardiography is only as good as the individual performing the examination and that the training, accreditation and continuing education of echocardiographers is essential to the effective functioning of a clinical service. Moreover there is an increasing drive for the accreditation of echocardiography laboratories and individual accreditation of echocardiographers is a central part of this process.

Sitting an accreditation examination is a daunting prospect for many trainee echocardiographers. There are numerous textbooks on echocardiography covering the range from basic to advanced imaging but few that provide specific preparation for examinations. In this book Sanjay Banypersad, Keith Pearce and their colleagues have set out to provide a revision aid based broadly on the current syllabus of the British Society for Echocardiography. Writing unambiguous multiple choice questions and selecting video cases relevant to clinical practice is far from easy and the authors and text reviewers have made strenuous efforts to ensure the accuracy and relevance of the content.

No book of this type is sufficient on its own to provide all the information required for individual accreditation but used in conjunction with one of the comprehensive echocardiography texts available it should be very useful to those preparing for examinations or simply wanting to refresh their knowledge.

Simon Ray, BSc, MD, FRCP, FACC, FESC
Consultant Cardiologist
Honorary Professor of Cardiology
University Hospitals of South Manchester
Manchester Academic Health Sciences Centre
Manchester, UK

Preface

There has been a vast expansion in the field of cardiac imaging in recent years. Coronary CT is now part of NICE guidance for low-risk ischaemic heart disease and cardiac MRI is increasingly favoured for certain pathologies. Echocardiography remains however of paramount importance in the cardiological assessment of patients. Its fundamental advantage lies in being widely available, cost-effective and easily portable without any appreciable reduction in picture quality. This has meant not only an increase in the number of studies being performed per year, but also in the specialty of the operator performing the studies. Emergency physicians and anaesthetists are now well versed in the application of echocardiography to critically ill patients in the resuscitation department, ICU or operating theatres.

It is important therefore that adherence to a quality standard is safeguarded to ensure that the patient receives a uniformly high standard of examination. There are a number of accreditation processes worldwide and this book is designed to broadly mimic the layout of the British Society of Echocardiography Transthoracic accreditation process, which currently comprises a written MCQ paper and a video section. This book has 8 chapters derived from the current syllabus and each chapter consists of 20 MCQ style questions each with 5 'True/False' stems, except the LV Assessment chapter which has 30 questions. Chapter 9 is comprised of 20 video cases each consisting of 4 or 5 questions with the option to pick one 'best-fit' answer from the given stems.

It is my hope that all candidates sitting a board exam or accreditation will find this book an invaluable revision aid and that those not sitting for accreditation will still nevertheless find it useful for their continued professional development.

Sanjay M. Banypersad

Acknowledgements

We would like to extend our gratitude to the following people for their time and effort spent in addition to their clinical duties, in order to peer-review all the material in this book.

Dr Simon Ray, Consultant Cardiologist, University Hospitals South Manchester NHS Foundation Trust, Wythenshawe Hospital, Southmoor Road, Manchester, UK.

Dr Nik Abidin, Consultant Cardiologist, Salford Royal NHS Foundation Trust, Salford Royal Hospital, Stott Lane, Salford, UK.

Miss Jane Lynch, Expert Cardiac Physiologist, University Hospitals South Manchester NHS Foundation Trust, Wythenshawe Hospital, Southmoor Road, Manchester, UK.

Dr Anna Herrey, Consultant in Cardiology, The Heart Hospital, 16–18 Westmoreland Street, London, UK.

Dr Ansuman Saha, Consultant Cardiologist, East Surrey Hospital, Canada Avenue, Redhill, Surrey, UK.

Dr Richard Bogle, Consultant Cardiologist, Epsom and St. Helier University Hospital NHS Trust, Wrythe Lane, Carshalton, Surrey, UK.

Dr Anita MacNab, Consultant Cardiologist, University Hospitals South Manchester NHS Foundation Trust, Wythenshawe Hospital, Southmoor Road, Manchester, UK.

Dr Bruce Irwin, SpR in Cardiology, University Hospitals South Manchester NHS Foundation Trust, Wythenshawe Hospital, Southmoor Road, Manchester, UK.

We are also grateful to all the echocardiographers and technicians in the echocardiography department at Wythenshawe Hospital and to the University Hospitals South Manchester NHS Foundation Trust for their permission to use the images and video files.

Sanjay M. Banypersad would also like to add a final vote of thanks to his parents and younger brother, Vishal, for their constant words of support and encouragement throughout.

Abbreviations

5-HT	5-Hydroxytryptamine
ACC	American College of Cardiology
ACHD	adult congenital heart disease
AHA	American Heart Association
AF	atrial fibrillation
AR	aortic regurgitation
ARVC	arrhythmogenic right ventricular cardiomyopathy
AS	aortic stenosis
ASD	atrial septal defect
AV	aortic valve
AVR	aortic valve replacement
AVSD	atrioventricular septal defects
BP	blood pressure
BSA	body surface area
BSE	British Society of Echocardiography
CAD	coronary artery disease
CRT	cardiac resynchronisation therapy
CSA	cross-sectional area
CT	computed tomography
CW	continuous wave
dB	decibel
DCM	dilated cardiomyopathy
dP	change in pressure
DSE	dobutamine stress echocardiogram
dT	change in time
dV	change in volume
ECG	electrocardiogram
E–F	not strictly an abbreviation – refers to anterior mitral leaflet movement on M-mode in the active and passive phase of transmitral flow
EF	ejection fraction
EPSS	E-point septal separation
ESC	European Society of Cardiology
HCM	hypertrophic cardiomyopathy
HOCM	hypertrophic obstructive cardiomyopathy

HR	heart rate
ICU	intensive care unit
IV	intravenous
IVC	inferior vena cava
IVCT	Isovolumetric contraction time
IVRT	Isovolumetric relaxation time
IVSd	interventricular septum in diastole
JVP	jugular venous pressure
LA	left atrium
LAD	left anterior descending
LBBB	left bundle branch block
LV	left ventricle
LVAD	left ventricular assist device
LVEDD	left ventricular end-diastolic dimension
LVEDP	left ventricular end-diastolic pressure
LVESD	left ventricular end-systolic dimension
LVH	left ventricular hypertrophy
LVIT	left ventricular inflow tract
LVOT	left ventricular outflow tract
MI	myocardial infarction
MS	mitral stenosis
MR	mitral regurgitation
MRI	magnetic resonance imaging
MV	mitral valve
MVP	mitral valve prolapse
MVR	mitral valve replacement
NICE	National Institute for Health and Clinical Excellence
PA	pulmonary artery
PDA	patent ductus arteriosus
PE	pulmonary embolism
PFO	patent foramen ovale
PISA	proximal isovelocity surface area
PPM	permanent pacemaker
PR	pulmonary regurgitation
PRF	pulse-resonance frequency
PS	pulmonary stenosis
PV	pulmonary valve
PW	pulsed wave
RA	right atrium
RBBB	right bundle branch block
RCA	right coronary artery
RCM	restrictive cardiomyopathy

ROA	regurgitant orifice area
RV	right ventricle
RVH	right ventricular hypertrophy
RVOT	right ventricular outflow tract
RWMA	regional wall motion abnormality
SLE	systemic lupus erythematosus
SV	stroke volume
SVC	superior vena cava
SVR	systemic vascular resistance
TAPSE	tricuspid annular plane systolic excursion
TB	tuberculosis
TOE	transoesophageal echocardiography
TR	tricuspid regurgitation
TTE	transthoracic echocardiography
TV	tricuspid valve
V	velocity
VSD	ventricular septal defect
VTI	velocity time integral

1 Basic Physics and Anatomy

QUESTIONS

For each question below, decide whether the answers provided are true or false.

1 The following is true of ultrasound waves:
   a. Propagate through medium like light
   b. Are part of the electromagnetic spectrum
   c. Loudness is measured in decibels
   d. The decibel scale shows a linear relationship with amplitude ratio
   e. Can be reflected but not refracted

2 The following are true of ultrasound waves during 2D echo:
   a. The optimal image is formed when the medium is perpendicular to the ultrasound beam
   b. The narrowest part of the beam (the focal zone) can be varied
   c. Side lobes are artefacts only found with phased-array transducers
   d. Structures smaller in diameter than the wavelength of the ultrasound beam may cause scattering of the beam
   e. Travel faster in blood than in bone

3 During standard TTE:
   a. Dropout occurs when there is parallel alignment of the beam with the tissue
   b. At a higher frequency, the ultrasound beam has a higher penetration depth
   c. Doppler studies are based on scattering of the ultrasound beam by red blood cells

Successful Accreditation in Echocardiography: A Self-Assessment Guide,
First Edition. Sanjay M. Banypersad and Keith Pearce.
© 2012 John Wiley & Sons, Ltd. Published 2012 by John Wiley & Sons, Ltd.

   d. The transmitted ultrasound waves are attenuated with
increasing mismatch in acoustic impedance

   e. Axial resolution degrades more than lateral resolution when
the depth is increased

4 The following are true of image resolution and artefacts:

   a. M-mode has excellent temporal resolution

   b. Prosthetic valves cause acoustic shadowing as well as
reverberations

   c. Tissue harmonic imaging improves endocardial border
definition but has no effect on valves

   d. High PRF can cause uncertainty due to range ambiguity

   e. Low aliasing velocities with colour Doppler can overestimate
regurgitation

5 During echocardiography, the following can be changed by the
operator:

   a. Impedance

   b. Focus

   c. Amplitude

   d. Wavelength

   e. PRF

6 Regarding the use of tissue Doppler imaging:

   a. It can be used to calculate myocardial tissue velocities

   b. It can give information on segmental LV function

   c. Unlike transmitral E and A velocities are, tissue Doppler
imaging-derived E' and A' waves are not preload dependent

   d. Gives a more accurate assessment of IVRT than transmitral
Doppler

   e. The heart's movement in the chest cavity can be a limitation
of the technique

7 When using M-mode to assess LV ejection fraction:

   a. May be inaccurate if the beam is oblique

   b. Results may not be indicative of overall function in ischaemic
heart disease

   c. End-systolic dimensions are usually measured on the R wave
of the ECG

   d. A fractional shortening of 30% can be normal

   e. The result is more accurate than EF derived using the
Simpson's method

8 Regarding PW Doppler, the following are true:
  a. Is subject to the Nyquist limit
  b. Has two dedicated crystals for sending and receiving
  c. Can measure velocities at varying depth
  d. Is used in tissue Doppler imaging
  e. More than one sample volume can be assessed at a time

9 Regarding continuous-wave Doppler, the following are true:
  a. Transmits and receives an impulse in sequence.
  b. Is useful in assessing mid-cavity step-ups in gradient
  c. Often aliases at high velocities
  d. Is limited in that it cannot separate individual velocities along the length of a beam
  e. Is useful when assessing peak aortic velocity

10 For a 5 MHz transducer at an angle of 60° to blood flow, the Doppler frequency shift is 10 kHz. The following are true:
  a. The wavelength is approximately 0.3 mm
  b. The maximum depth is 2–3 cm
  c. The blood velocity is approximately 3 m/s
  d. Lowering the transducer frequency to 1 MHz increases maximum depth to 20 cm
  e. Optimal accuracy occurs with the Doppler cursor perpendicular to the direction of flow

11 In standard 2D echocardiography of a patient lying in the left lateral position:
  a. The atrial septum is best visualised in the apical 4-chamber view
  b. In the apical 4-chamber view, tilting the ultrasound beam posteriorly reveals the 5-chamber view
  c. In the parasternal long-axis view, tilting the beam infero-medially reveals the RV inflow
  d. In the parasternal long axis view, the normal LA is ≤4.5 cm in men
  e. Coronary arteries can sometimes be seen in the parasternal short-axis view

12 Regarding the parasternal short-axis view:
  a. The most posterior of the aortic valve cusps is the non-coronary cusp
  b. The mitral valve leaflets are clearly seen

    c. It is a useful view for detecting PV abnormalities

    d. It is a useful view for calculating PA pressure

    e. Eccentric jets of regurgitant aortic or mitral valves can be clearly demonstrated

13 In the apical 4-chamber view:

    a. The right ventricular wall is thinner than that of the LV

    b. A septal 'knuckle' is often seen in elderly people

    c. The Chiari network may be seen in the LA

    d. Rotating to the apical 3-chamber view reveals the inferior wall

    e. Rotating to the apical 2-chamber view shows the aortic valve

14 Regarding spectral Doppler signals:

    a. The normal mitral E wave is greater than the A wave in young people

    b. Peak aortic velocity of >2 m/s can be normal with some prosthetic valves

    c. In AF, an average of at least five consecutive signals should be taken

    d. CW Doppler is usually needed for high velocities to avoid aliasing

    e. A fast sweep-speed is required to assess for respiratory variation

15 The following relationships between structures is true in the parasternal long axis:

    a. The left coronary cusp of the aortic valve is anterior

    b. A fibrous band separates the anterior mitral valve leaflet and the aortic root

    c. In the RV inflow view, the anterior and posterior tricuspid valve leaflets are seen

    d. The moderator band can be seen in the RV

    e. The nodules of Arantius are features of the mitral valve

16 The following parameters would not affect frame rate:

    a. Increasing the depth

    b. Increasing the sector size

    c. Increasing the line density

    d. Increasing the transmit frequency

    e. Decreasing the sector size

17 The type of filter used for tissue Doppler imaging is a:
  a. High-pass filter
  b. Band-pass filter
  c. Low-pass filter
  d. Reject filter
  e. Notch filter

18 Dobutamine stress echo:
  a. Cannot be used to detect myocardial viability
  b. Can be used to diagnose CAD
  c. Is more sensitive and specific than exercise stress testing
  d. Can be used to predict anaesthetic risk for major surgery
  e. Is usually performed using agitated saline contrast

19 Harmonic imaging:
  a. Was developed to improve endocardial definition
  b. Uses a transmit frequency equal to the receive frequency
  c. Enhances the detection of transpulmonary contrast
  d. Makes valvular structures appear thicker
  e. Should not be used when making Doppler recordings

20 The following statements are true:
  a. Absorption is the transfer of ultrasound energy to the tissue during propagation
  b. Acoustic impedance is the product of tissue density and the propagation velocity through it
  c. Shifting the zero velocity baseline may eliminate aliasing in the pulsed-wave Doppler mode
  d. Shadowing results in the presence of echoes directly behind a strong echo reflector
  e. A longitudinal wave is a cyclic disturbance in which the energy propagation is parallel to the direction of particle motion

Basic Physics and Anatomy

ANSWERS

1 a. F
   b. F
   c. T
   d. F
   e. F

Visible light is part of the electromagnetic spectrum and is propagated as a transverse waves. Sound is not part of the electromagnetic spectrum and is propagated as longitudinal waves, with oscillations parallel to the direction of propagation. Loudness is measured in decibels and the scale shows a logarithmic relationship to amplitude ratio i.e. dB = 20 log (V/R) (where V represents acoustic pressure and R is a reference value). Ultrasound waves can be both reflected and refracted, the latter being responsible for false images in aberrant locations.

2 a. T
   b. T
   c. F
   d. T
   e. F

Reflection of ultrasound waves (and therefore imaging) is optimal when the tissue interface is perpendicular with the ultrasound beam. The normal ultrasound beam from a transducer of diameter D, travels through an aperture and has an initial columnar near zone; beyond this, there is divergence of the beam, according to sin θ = 1.22λ/D, which causes image degradation. However, the transducer face can be altered to become, for example, more concave, changing the position of the narrowest point of the beam so that image resolution is greater – this is the focal zone and it is variable. Side lobes are beams dispersed laterally to the main beam leading to image artefact and are common to all transducers; grating lobes are specific to phased-array transducers. Scattering is caused by structures smaller than the wavelength of the ultrasound beam. Structures larger in wavelength cause reflection or refraction. The propagation velocity in bone is double that of blood.

3 a. T
 b. F
 c. T
 d. T
 e. F

Parallel alignment causes very little of the ultrasound beam to be reflected back to the transducer, causing image dropout; this is typically seen of the atrial septum in apical 4-chamber view. A higher frequency produces higher image resolution but decreases penetration depth. The wavelength of ultrasound is 0.2–1 mm, whereas that of a red cell is about 7–10 μm, hence as stated above, red blood cells are effective scatterers and form the principle of Doppler flow studies. Air has high acoustic impedance, so any air between the transducer and the body causes a significant acoustic impedance mismatch and therefore attenuation of the transmitted beam; attenuation can also affect the reflected beam. Axial resolution is relatively unchanged with increasing depth because the beam remains parallel to the tissues. However, lateral resolution decreases because beam width increases due to divergence.

4 a. T
 b. T
 c. F
 d. T
 e. T

M-mode does have excellent temporal resolution and is often used to assess high-speed motion such as mitral valve leaflet fluttering. Prosthetic valves can cause reverberation and acoustic shadowing beyond the valve image. Harmonics improve border definition but also make valves appear thicker, thus standard imaging should always be used in conjunction with harmonics. High PRF is useful to detect very high velocities, but range ambiguity means that the depth at which that velocity occurs could be located at any one of several points along the insonating beam. Low aliasing velocities cause distinct colour changes at lower velocities than normal, making the degree of regurgitation seem higher than it actually is.

5 a. F
  b. T
  c. T
  d. F
  e. T

Impedance is a property of the tissue itself. Wavelength is usually fixed, and since velocity is constant through a given medium, PRF can be altered to produce varying depth. Amplitude is altered through gain and the focus can be varied as explained above (see answer to Question 4)

6 a. T
  b. T
  c. T
  d. F
  e. T

Tissue Doppler imaging can assess myocardial tissue velocities and indeed, the myocardial velocity gradient between 2 positions on the ventricle; it can therefore be very useful for assessing segmental motion and function. Because myocardial velocities rather than blood flow velocities are measured, they are less preload dependent. However, IVRT is best measured with conventional PW Doppler as myocardial movement does not necessarily correlate with valve opening and closure.

7 a. T
  b. T
  c. F
  d. T
  e. F

M-mode has excellent time resolution and endocardial border motion is well imaged. A very oblique beam will overestimate cavity size and underestimate function as displacement is at an angle to the insonating beam. Maximal displacement measurement will occur when the beam is perpendicular to the chamber. Regional wall motion abnormalities are common is ischaemic heart disease and a large apical infarct with preserved basal segments would overestimate LV function with M-mode. End-diastolic dimensions are measured on the R wave and the normal range for fractional shortening is 25–45%. Simpson's method is a more accurate measure of EF as a number of segments across the LV cavity are included.

8 a. T
  b. F
  c. T
  d. T
  e. T

Pulsed-wave Doppler sends out a signal from one crystal and waits for it to return before sending out another. The sample depth is fixed by the operator and any Doppler shift caused to the initial transmitted signal by blood flow is detected by the transducer on the return signal and this is displayed on the spectral analysis. The Nyquist limit is the maximum velocity that can be assessed by PW Doppler at a given frequency and depth. Exceeding this causes aliasing. Sample depth can be altered by the operator to measure velocities at varying depths and using high pulse-repetition frequencies, more than one depth can be sampled at any one time. Tissue Doppler uses PW Doppler with different ranges set for velocity measurement.

9 a. F
  b. F
  c. F
  d. T
  e. T

Continuous-wave Doppler has one crystal constantly transmitting and one crystal constantly receiving signals and is therefore not subject to aliasing or the Nyquist limit. It can only measure all velocities across the entire length of a beam and not separate them out and is therefore not useful for assessing mid-cavity gradients. Peak aortic velocity is often the highest velocity within the heart and CW Doppler is therefore used primarily for acquiring this parameter.

10 a. T
  b. F
  c. T
  d. F
  e. F

Wavelength is calculated by $c = \lambda f$, with c being speed of sound in blood, which remains constant at 1540 m/s. For a transducer frequency of 5 MHz, the wavelength is 0.31 mm. The maximum depth is limited to approximately 200 wavelengths, thus maximum depth in this example is 6 cm. Blood velocity is calculated using the formula $V = c(\Delta f) \div 2\,F_T(\cos\theta)$ where Δf is change in frequency and F_T is transducer frequency. In this example, the blood velocity works out as around 3 m/s. Transducer frequency of 1 MHz produces a maximum depth of 30 cm and optimal accuracy with Doppler should be directly in line with the direction of flow, not perpendicular to it (which is required for image display from ultrasound waves).

11 a. F
  b. F
  c. T
  d. T
  e. T

The atrial septum is prone to dropout in the 4-chamber view and is often best seen in the subcostal view. In the apical 4-chamber view, tilting the beam anteriorly will produce the 5-chamber view. In the parasternal long-axis view, tilting the beam inferiorly and medially will bring in the RV inflow tract whereas tilting it superiorly (i.e. towards the left shoulder) can reveal the PV. The normal LA is <4.5 cm in men. The left main and right coronary arteries can sometimes be seen in the parasternal short-axis view.

12 a. T
  b. T
  c. T
  d. T
  e. T

All three aortic valve cusps can be seen in the parasternal short-axis view; the non-coronary cusp is the most posterior. At the mitral valve level, the anterior and posterior leaflet can be clearly seen and at the aortic level, the PV can be seen, usually near the junction of the left and non-coronary cusps. PA pressure can be calculated from the TR jet, which can also often be seen in this view and in many other views.

13 a. T
  b. T
  c. F
  d. F
  e. F

The right ventricular wall is normally thinner than the LV and a septal 'knuckle' or prominent septal bulge is a common finding in elderly people, usually of no clinical significance. The Chiari network is found in the RA. The apical 3-chamber view reveals the posterior wall, anteroseptal wall and the aortic valve; the 2-chamber view shows the mitral valve, anterior wall and inferior wall.

14 a. T
   b. T
   c. T
   d. T
   e. F

The transmitral E wave is usually higher than the A wave in young patients with normal hearts, indicating a highly compliant LV. Peak velocity across a prosthetic aortic valve can be 2–3 m/s. At least 5–10 signals should be recorded in AF due to variability of flow with the irregularity of each heart beat. CW Doppler is generally needed for high velocities as PW Doppler leads to aliasing. A slow sweep-speed is required to accurately assess respiratory variation across mitral or tricuspid Doppler.

15 a. F
   b. F
   c. F
   d. T
   e. F

The right coronary cusp is anterior and the non-coronary cusp is posterior. The anterior mitral valve leaflet and aortic root are in fibrous continuity, they are not separated. The anterior and septal leaflets of the tricuspid are seen in the RV inflow view and the moderator band can be seen in the RV. The nodules of Arantius are features of the aortic valve.

16 a. F
   b. F
   c. F
   d. T
   e. F

Altering the depth will reduce or increase frame rates due to time taken for the ultrasound to reach the required depth and return to the transmission point. Shallow depth = high frame rate. Line density will also directly affect frame rates. An increase or decrease of transmission frequency within either fundamental or harmonic imaging modalities has no direct impact on the overall frame rate.

17 a. F
   b. F
   c. T
   d. F
   e. F

High-pass filters remove low-frequency signals, which make up the basis of tissue motion, therefore a low-pass filter is utilised to enable the high-frequency signals to be removed allowing concentration on the signal returned from the myocardium.

18 a. F
   b. T
   c. T
   d. T
   e. F

The major purpose of DSE includes the detection of myocardial viability and ischaemia in the presence of coronary disease. Low-dose dobutamine studies help to diagnose the presence/absence of viable myocardium; high-dose dobutamine helps demonstrate the presence/absence of myocardial ischaemia due to CAD. DSE is more sensitive and specific than exercise stress testing. Preoperative risk can be assessed in patients undergoing major non-cardiac surgery. Transpulmonary contrast is utilised during DSE due to its ability to cross the pulmonary capillary system.

19 a. F
   b. F
   c. T
   d. T
   e. F

The development of harmonic imaging was in association with the development of transpulmonary contrast to promote resonance of the contrast media and prevent destruction of contrast in the near field. The transmit frequency is half of the received frequency although care should be made due to poor image quality in both the near and far field regions when using harmonic imaging. The valves do appear thicker when utilising harmonic frequency imaging and the endocardial border can often be seen more clearly although these are coincidental findings from the technology development. Doppler recordings are not affected when using harmonic 2D imaging.

20 a. T
   b. T
   c. T
   d. F
   e. T

Absorption is indeed the transfer of ultrasound energy to the tissue during propagation. Acoustic impedance is calculated by tissue density × propagation velocity through that tissue. Shifting the zero velocity baseline down can reduce higher velocities from aliasing on the pulse-wave spectral Doppler display up to a limit. A strong echo reflector will not allow any ultrasound through it and little or no echo will appear behind the reflector. A longitudinal wave propagates energy parallel to the direction of motion.

2 The Aortic Valve

QUESTIONS

For each question below, decide whether the answers provided are true or false.

1 The following are true when performing echocardiography in AS:
   a. Systolic separation of the leaflets of more than 15 mm reliably excludes severe AS
   b. Maximum gradient at Doppler correlates exactly with peak-to-peak gradient at cardiac catheterisation
   c. Valve area is most commonly assessed by direct planimetry in the parasternal short axis
   d. Pressure gradients from Doppler studies are independent of flow rate
   e. Mean pressure gradient in AS is approximately $2.4v^2$

2 The following are true regarding abnormalities of the aortic valve:
   a. Doming leaflets with commissural fusion suggests a rheumatic aetiology
   b. Bicuspid valve is the commonest cause of AS
   c. A bicuspid valve can exhibit bowing or doming similar to MS
   d. Identification of the number of leaflets should occur in diastole
   e. All of the above

3 The following can aid differentiation of true valvular stenosis from fixed supra- or subvalvular obstruction:
   a. CW Doppler
   b. PW Doppler
   c. Pedoff probe

Successful Accreditation in Echocardiography: A Self-Assessment Guide,
First Edition. Sanjay M. Banypersad and Keith Pearce.
© 2012 John Wiley & Sons, Ltd. Published 2012 by John Wiley & Sons, Ltd.

    d. TOE

    e. Tissue Doppler

4 When performing calculations and measurements in AS:

    a. In the presence of LV dysfunction, dobutamine challenge at low dose may be useful

    b. The LVOT diameter should be measured on the R wave of the ECG

    c. The presence of AR may increase the transaortic pressure gradient due to increased flow

    d. The stand-alone CW Doppler probe is less accurate than the standard imaging probe when measuring peak aortic velocities

    e. 3D echo has no role to play in the assessment of AS

5 When assessing AS:

    a. Peak aortic velocity of 4.5 m/s is consistent with severe AS

    b. LVH is a recognised association

    c. A valve area of 1.2 cm^2 may indicate severe stenosis if LV dysfunction is present

    d. The stand-alone CW Doppler probe can only be used in the apical position to quantify the peak velocity

    e. The degree of tricuspid regurgitation is a determinant for intervention

6 With normal LV function, the following suggest moderate AS:

    a. Valve area of 0.8 cm^2

    b. A mean gradient of 45 mmHg

    c. A peak velocity of 2.7 m/s

    d. Late peaking of the CW Doppler jet

    e. A wide pulse pressure

7 With regard to the AV:

    a. Diagnosis of a bicuspid AV is only possible on M-Mode

    b. Lambl's excrescences are normal variants

    c. Nodules of Arantius are not normal variants

    d. In the parasternal short-axis view, the non-coronary cusp is anatomically closest to the PA

    e. The LVOT should be measured approximately 1 cm below the valve at the point where PW Doppler would be measured.

8 The following statements are true regarding the AV:
  a. Has 2 papillary muscles
  b. Can calcify in a process similar to atherosclerosis
  c. Can have up to four leaflets
  d. A valve area of up to 4 cm^2 would be considered normal
  e. With increasing stenosis of the valve, wall stress remains constant until LV failure occurs

9 You are called to ICU to perform an echo on a patient with known AS. The LVOT velocity is 0.8 m/s and LVOT diameter is 2.4 cm. CW Doppler reveals a mean gradient of 48 mmHg, transaortic VTI of 70 cm and systolic ejection time of 320 ms. The following are true:
  a. Peak aortic velocity is 3.5 m/s
  b. AV area is approximately 0.8 cm^2
  c. Stroke volume cannot be calculated from the data above
  d. SVR is 364 dynes.s.cm^{-5}
  e. Cardiac output cannot be calculated from the data above

10 The following are true of bicuspid AVs:
  a. Can be familial
  b. Are found in 70–80% of coarctations
  c. Are a recognised cause of AR as well as AS
  d. Bicuspid PVs are recognised associations
  e. In the parasternal short axis, the closure line can be eccentric

11 The following are recognised causes of AR:
  a. Aortic dissection
  b. Endocarditis
  c. Hypertension
  d. Marfan's syndrome
  e. Ehlers–Danlos syndrome

12 The following aetiological associations are recognised in AR:
  a. Calcified aortic valve suggests myxomatous disease
  b. Leaflet perforation suggests endocarditis as the most likely aetiology
  c. Aortic root dilatation suggests Marfan's syndrome as the most likely cause
  d. Thickened leaflets suggests myxomatous disease
  e. A false 'mass' effect can be seen with thickened leaflets in the short-axis view

13 The following findings are consistent with severe AS:
   a. Peak pressure drop >64 mmHg
   b. Mean pressure drop >40 mmHg
   c. Presence of LVH
   d. Aortic valve area <1.0 cm^2
   e. Calcified AV (three cusps)

14 When performing TTE in patients with AR:
   a. Increased E-point septal separation is only seen because of LV dilatation
   b. Motion abnormality in the anterior MV leaflet similar to HOCM is seen
   c. Reverse doming of the MV may be seen
   d. Functional MS may be seen with very eccentric jets
   e. Type A dissections do not cause AR

15 The following suggest moderate AR:
   a. Regurgitant volume of 45 ml/beat
   b. Jet width of 40% LVOT area
   c. Pressure half time of 350 ms
   d. Regurgitant orifice area of 0.4 cm^2
   e. Peak forward velocity 3 m/s

16 The following are true regarding anatomy of the AV and root:
   a. In Marfan's syndrome, patients should only be considered for root replacement when aortic root dilatation of ≥5.5 cm occurs
   b. In the parasternal short-axis view, the non-coronary cusp is closer to the LA than the right coronary cusp
   c. The left mainstem coronary artery can sometimes be seen originating close to the left coronary cusp
   d. Sinotubular junction measurement is usually greater than that of the sinus of valsalva
   e. The valve is usually not visualised in the suprasternal view

17 The following suggest severe AR:
   a. Vena contracta of 0.8 cm
   b. Regurgitant fraction of 45%
   c. CW Doppler density equal to forward flow signal intensity
   d. Holodiastolic flow reversal in the descending aorta in the suprasternal view
   e. Peak transaortic pressure gradient by Bernoulli equation of 75 mmHg

18 The following statements are true regarding AR:
  a. Moderate AR should be followed up with yearly echo scans
  b. Acute severe AR can cause equalisation of LV and aortic end-diastolic pressures
  c. Chronic severe AR produces a low diastolic aortic pressure
  d. Is associated with ankylosing spondylitis
  e. Regurgitant volumes in AR can only be calculated if the stroke volumes at 2 different sites are known

19 The following are true of aortic dissection:
  a. Hypertension is a risk factor
  b. Type B aortic dissections do not involve the ascending aorta
  c. Can cause ST elevation MIs if the dissection involves the right coronary ostium
  d. Type A dissections carry significant mortality without early surgery
  e. Are well recognised after high-velocity, road traffic accidents

20 The following are true regarding abnormalities of the AV and root:
  a. Quadricuspid valves are recognised
  b. Kawasaki's disease is associated with aortic aneurysms
  c. A sinus of valsalva aneurysm at the non-coronary cusp would protrude into the RV
  d. Severe AR is a contraindication for an intra-aortic balloon pump
  e. Syphilis can cause aneurysms of the aorta

The Aortic Valve

ANSWERS

1 a. T
   b. F
   c. F
   d. F
   e. T

Although leaflet opening of <15 mm does not distinguish between mild, moderate or severe stenosis, opening of >15 mm reliably excludes severe stenosis. Catheter pullback measures peak-to-peak pressure difference between the LV and the aorta. These pressures do not occur at the same point in time. CW Doppler measures peak instantaneous pressure difference that is greater than the peak-to-peak difference. This explains in part why transaortic pressure gradients calculated at catheterisation are lower than those calculated from Doppler. Direct planimetry of the AV is difficult to reproduce accurately because of the complex nature of its tricuspid appearance, thus Doppler provides the best functional assessment of valve area. Pressure gradients are affected by flow rate, such that severe AS with LV dysfunction may generate a moderate gradient even though stenosis is severe. Maximum pressure gradient is calculated by $\Delta P_{max} = 4v^2$ whereas mean gradient is ΔP_{mean}, which approximates as $2.4v^2$.

2 a. T
   b. F
   c. T
   d. T
   e. F

Doming leaflets with commissural fusion does suggest a rheumatic aetiology; the valves can be trileaflet, appearing functionally bicuspid because of fusion along the commissures. Calcific disease is the commonest cause of AS. Bicuspid valves may exhibit a bowing or doming appearance on echo, similar to MS. Identification of the number of leaflets should occur in systole as the leaflets of bicuspid valves are unequal in size, and raphe in the larger leaflet can, when closed, give the erroneous appearance of a TV.

3 a. F
  b. T
  c. F
  d. T
  e. F

CW Doppler displays only the peak velocity across the profile, therefore the anatomical point of step-up in velocity in the LVOT cannot be determined. PW Doppler allows velocities to be measured at a specific point in the LVOT and aorta using the sampling volume. The stand-alone Pedoff probe will identify the peak aortic velocity but will not delineate the anatomical location and is not therefore useful in distinguishing between true stenosis and other causes. TOE will allow accurate visualisation of structures like sub-aortic membranes. Tissue Doppler measures low velocity large amplitude movements such as mitral annular motion in assessment of diastolic dysfunction; it has no role in identifying the level of obstruction.

4 a. T
  b. F
  c. T
  d. F
  e. F

In LV dysfunction, there is a low-flow rate through the AV, resulting in a lower gradient and apparently less severe stenosis. Infusion of dobutamine augments cardiac output and if the valve is truly severely stenosed, the peak aortic velocity will increase as a larger volume of blood is forced through an unchanged orifice per unit time. The LVOT diameter should be measured in mid-systole. Coexisting AR results in increased transaortic volume flow, thereby increasing peak pressure gradient. However, valve areas calculated using the continuity equation are still accurate as $CSA_{LVOT} \times VTI_{LVOT}$ is still equal to aortic stroke volume. The stand-alone CW Doppler is more accurate than the imaging probe for peak aortic velocity measurement as it has a smaller area and allows better alignment with the direction of flow. 3D LV volumes can be used to calculate stroke volume. This may be more accurate than stroke volume derived from measurements of the LVOT diameter and PW Doppler.

5 a. T
  b. T
  c. F
  d. F
  e. F

A peak velocity above 4 m/s suggests severe AS. LVH is commonly seen as the LV adapts to overcome the obstructive valve. In low-flow AS, the peak pressure gradient may be low but valve area calculations (by continuity equation) are still accurate. Therefore a valve area of 1.2 cm^2 would be in the moderate category. The stand-alone CW Doppler probe can be used in the suprasternal and right sternal edge. The degree of tricuspid regurgitation is irrelevant when determining the necessity for AVR.

6 a. F
  b. F
  c. F
  d. F
  e. F

A valve area of 0.8 cm^2 and a mean gradient of 45 mmHg represent severe AS. A peak gradient of 45 mmHg would represent moderate AS. A peak velocity of 2.7 m/s is in the mild category, moderate would be in the region of 3–4 m/s. Late peaking of the CW jet suggests HOCM and has no bearing in determining severity of AS. A wide pulse pressure is seen in AR, not AS.

7 a. F
  b. T
  c. F
  d. F
  e. T

Assessment of the number of cusps of the AV should occur in systole, as a bicuspid valve may appear tricuspid in diastole due to prominent raphe. This usually shows an eccentric closure line but can be seen as a central closure line on M-Mode. Lambl's excrescences are small mobile filaments on the LV aspect of the aortic valve and are normal variants. Nodules of Arantius are enlargements of the normal thickening present on the free edge of all the cusps and are also normal variants. In the parasternal short-axis view, the non-coronary cusp is closest to the RA and LA; the left coronary cusp is seen closest to the PA. To reproduce reliability and accuracy, the LVOT indeed should be measured 1 cm below the valve at the point where PW Doppler would be measured.

8 a. F
 b. T
 c. T
 d. T
 e. T

The AV supports its own structure and does not have papillary muscles. It commonly calcifies in a process similar to atherosclerosis, indeed there is ongoing work assessing the use of statin therapy in slowing progression of stenosis. It is most commonly tricuspid but up to four leaflets have been recognised. The normal aortic valve area is 2–4 cm^2 and wall stress is related to pressure overload (P) and wall thickness (Th) by : wall stress $\approx$ (R/Th) $\times$ P, where R is the ventricular radius.

9 a. F
 b. T
 c. F
 d. T
 e. T

Peak aortic velocity can be derived knowing the mean gradient = approximately 2.4 v^2. In this example, it is 4.5 m/s. Knowing this, AV area can be approximated using the velocities instead of VTIs in the continuity equation, thus yielding a valve area of approximately 0.8 cm^2. Multiplying 0.8 by 70 (i.e. VTI$_{aortic}$) gives a stroke volume of 56 ml. SVR can be calculated: SVR = (1.33 × mean pressure gradient × systolic ejection time) ÷ stroke volume, which in this example gives an SVR of 364 dynes.s.cm^{-5}. Cardiac output cannot be calculated unless the pulse rate or R–R interval on an ECG is known.

10 a. T
 b. T
 c. T
 d. T
 e. T

Bicuspid aortic valves are prevalent in 1–2% of the population and are often familial. It is commonly found associated with coarctations of the aorta and dilated aortic roots. Both AR and AS are recognised, as are bicuspid PVs though the latter are rare. TVs have central closure lines whereas bicuspid valves generally have eccentric closure lines.

11 a. T
   b. T
   c. T
   d. T
   e. T
All are recognised causes. Rheumatic and calcific valve diseases are also recognised causes.

12 a. F
   b. T
   c. F
   d. T
   e. T
Calcified valves suggest primary calcific disease or previous rheumatic disease as the causative aetiology. Leaflet perforation is typical of endocarditis as is malcoaptation due to vegetations. Aortic root dilatation is commonly caused by hypertension; Marfan's syndrome and rheumatoid arthritis are not the most likely cause. Thickened, redundant leaflets are typical of myxomatous disease. Redundant leaflets sag in diastole, distorting the normal crown shape such that a leaflet is seen fully face on, giving the erroneous appearance of an ill-defined mass.

13 a. T
   b. T
   c. F
   d. T
   e. F
BSE guidelines currently state that severe AS occurs when the peak pressure drop is >64 mmHg and mean pressure drop is >40 mmHg. The presence of LVH does not necessarily indicate the need for intervention. An AV area of <1.0 cm^2 suggests severe AS and the presence of AV calcification may suggest aetiology but does not mandate surgery on its own.

14 a. F
   b. F
   c. T
   d. T
   e. F
Increased EPSS is seen because of the restriction in opening of the anterior MV leaflet due to the aortic regurgitant jet. High-frequency

fluttering of the anterior mitral leaflet can be seen in AR, whereas systolic anterior motion of the anterior mitral leaflet is usually associated with HOCM. Reverse doming of the anterior mitral leaflet can be seen in AR corresponding to the location of the regurgitant jet. Functional MS may be seen if MV opening is severely restricted, producing the characteristic Austin–Flint murmur. Type A aortic dissections involve the ascending aorta and may cause AR by either annular dilatation or leaflet disruption. Type B aortic dissections involve only the descending aorta and do not cause AR.

15 a. T
  b. T
  c. T
  d. F
  e. F

Moderate AR is defined by a regurgitant volume of 30–60 ml/beat, a jet width of 25–65% the LVOT area and a pressure half time of 200–500 ms. A regurgitant orifice area of $0.4 \, cm^2$ represents severe AR and the peak velocity does not feature in the classification of severity of AR.

16 a. F
  b. T
  c. T
  d. F
  e. T

Patients with Marfan's syndrome should be considered for root replacement when aortic root diameter is ≥4.5 cm. In the parasternal short-axis view, the non-coronary cusp is closer to the LA whereas the right coronary cusp is closer to the RV. The left mainstem can be seen originating close to the left coronary cusp. The sinus of valsalva measurement is usually the greater of the two. The aortic valve is not seen in the suprasternal view, which is mainly to assess flow reversal in severe AR.

17 a. T
  b. F
  c. T
  d. T
  e. F

Vena contracta of 0.3–0.6 cm represents moderate AR whereas >0.6 cm would be considered severe AR, as would a regurgitant fraction of >50%. A very dense signal jet equal to forward flow through the valve is in keeping with a severe jet of AR and holodiastolic flow reversal seen in the descending aorta is also considered in keeping with severe AR, although can occasionally be seen in moderate AR. Peak transaortic pressure gradient can be affected by the presence of AR (as flow across the aortic valve is increased) but is not a determinant of the severity of AR.

18 a. T
  b. T
  c. T
  d. T
  e. F

A finding of moderate AR should prompt annual follow-up scans to assess progression. In acute AR, there is no time for LV compliance to alter, leaving end-diastolic pressures very high, occasionally as high as aortic end-diastolic pressures. In chronic severe AR, pressure half times are very short, so aortic pressures fall quickly in diastole. Considering that LV compliance has adapted over time, the regurgitation is virtually unimpeded and aortic pressures drop very low in diastole. AR is frequently seen in ankylosing spondylitis. Unlike MR, regurgitant volumes in severe AR can be calculated from the proximal descending aorta, where the forward flow and stroke volume can be calculated, as well as the retrograde regurgitant jet.

19 a. T
  b. T
  c. T
  d. T
  e. T

Hypertension and Marfan's syndrome are risk factors for aortic dissection. Type B dissections involve only the descending aorta, whereas type A dissections may involve both ascending and descending aorta. Dissections involving the right coronary ostium can cause inferior ST elevation on an ECG – thrombolysis in these situations can be catastrophic. Type B dissections can often be conservatively managed but type A dissections carry a mortality of around 1% per h within the first 48 h. Although not common, aortic dissections are well recognised after road traffic accidents due to the shearing forces invoked within the thorax due to sudden loss of momentum.

20 a. T
   b. F
   c. F
   d. T
   e. T

Quadricuspid valves are rare but recognised. Kawasaki's disease generally causes aneurysms of the coronary arteries, particularly in children; Takayasu's disease can cause aortic aneurysms. A sinus of valsalva aneurysm at the non-coronary cusp would protrude into the RA not the RV. Severe AR is a contraindication to an intra-aortic balloon pump and is likely to overload the LV further if inserted. Syphilitic aortitis is a recognised complication of syphilis leading to aortic dilatation and aneurysms.

3 Left Ventricular Assessment

QUESTIONS

For each question below, decide whether the answers provided are true or false.

1 The following associations are recognised:
   a. Fabry's disease may produce a binary appearance of the endocardium
   b. Amyloidosis produces speckling of the myocardium
   c. Systolic anterior motion of the MV and HOCM
   d. Global dilatation and Tako–Tsubo cardiomyopathy
   e. Myocarditis and TV dysplasia

2 Finding LVH on echo would be consistent with which of the following diagnoses:
   a. Acute anterior MI
   b. HCM
   c. DCM
   d. Hypertension
   e. RCM

3 The following may be found in diastolic dysfunction:
   a. Transmitral E:A ratio of >1
   b. Transmitral E:A ratio of <1
   c. Tissue Doppler E/E' of <5
   d. Tissue Doppler E/E' of >10
   e. All of the above

Successful Accreditation in Echocardiography: A Self-Assessment Guide,
First Edition. Sanjay M. Banypersad and Keith Pearce.
© 2012 John Wiley & Sons, Ltd. Published 2012 by John Wiley & Sons, Ltd.

4 The following would be in keeping with mild–moderate diastolic dysfunction:

    a. Prolonged deceleration time

    b. Diastolic > systolic flow in the pulmonary veins

    c. Reversed transmitral Doppler E:A ratio

    d. Normal or increased isovolumic relaxation time

    e. Prominent atrial reversal in pulmonary venous flow Doppler

5 Normal LV systolic function:

    a. Shows a slight variation (<20%) in transmitral flow during respiration

    b. Can be affected by preload as well as afterload

    c. Is suggested by a cardiac output of 5–8 l/min at rest

    d. Shows a rapid pressure rise in early systole in the Doppler aortic flow signal

    e. Shows a long isovolumic contraction time in the Doppler aortic flow signal

6 The following are true regarding diastolic dysfunction:

    a. The change in volume : change in pressure ratio (dV/dP) represents LV compliance

    b. The change in pressure : change in volume ratio (dP/dV) represents LV stiffness

    c. Ventricular relaxation is a passive process

    d. LA filling does not increase with inspiration

    e. In severe diastolic dysfunction, the majority of LV filling occurs early in diastole

7 The presence of the following might reduce diastolic flow from LA to LV:

    a. Pericardial disease

    b. Atrial fibrillation

    c. Bradycardia

    d. Dehydration

    e. MR

8 A 63-year-old man presents with chest pain and hypotension to A&E. Echocardiography reveals: infero-posterior hypokinesia, moderate MR, time interval between 1 m/s to 3 m/s on MR jet = 40 ms, LVEDD 6.3 cm, LVESD 4.9 cm. He is in sinus rhythm. Which of the following are true:

    a. dP/dT = 800 mmHg/s

    b. The fractional shortening is approximately 40%

   c. LV systolic function is likely to be preserved

   d. The patient has likely had an LAD territory MI

   e. MR is a recognised complication of posterior MIs

9 You are called to perform an urgent echo on the coronary care unit. The patient is in sinus rhythm with a HR 90 bpm and BP 90/50 mmHg. His echo reveals: antero-apical hypokinesia with an ejection fraction 50% measured using M-mode, LVOT diameter 2.8 cm, VTI$_{LVOT}$ is 8 cm. Which of the following are true:

   a. The LV end-diastolic volume is approximately 100 ml

   b. The cardiac output is approximately 4.4 l/min

   c. The patient has likely had an LAD territory MI

   d. The patient has coexisting AS but not severe

   e. Apical VSDs are a recognised complication

10 In normal LV function:

   a. LV midwall fibres are orientated longitudinally

   b. Long-axis function declines with age, whereas short-axis function is relatively preserved

   c. The endocardium moves faster than the epicardium

   d. If severe MR is present, colour M-mode of the MR jet should produce a slope of 45°

   e. Pulmonary vein Doppler flow should show a systolic > diastolic pattern

11 A 53-year-old lady has an echo for exertional breathlessness. The parasternal long-axis view reveals: septum 1.5 cm, posterior wall 1.4 cm, LA volume 60 ml. The 4-chamber view reveals the transmitral E wave 1.02 m/s and A wave 0.98 m/s. The IVRT is normal. Which of the following are true:

   a. There is severe LVH

   b. The LA is mildly dilated

   c. The patient likely has moderate diastolic dysfunction even though IVRT is normal

   d. E/E′ velocities <5 would be expected

   e. The deceleration time is likely to be <100 ms

12 A 43-year-old hypertensive man has an echo. His BP is 182/100. In the parasternal long axis, the septum is 2.5 cm, posterior wall 2.4 cm, aortic root 4 cm. In the 4-chamber view, apical thickness is 2.4 cm, there is moderate AR with peak regurgitant velocity of 4.2 m/s and maximum forward flow across aortic valve of

2.5 m/s. PW reveals peak LVOT velocity of 2 m/s and a mid-cavity velocity of 1.5 m/s. Which of the following are true:
a. There is significant LVH.
b. The step up in mid-cavity gradient suggests the diagnosis is HCM
c. The patient requires aortic valve and root replacement
d. The LVEDP is about 30 mmHg
e. Severe hypertensive disease is present

13 The following are recognised causes of RCM:
a. Amyloidosis
b. Haemochromatosis
c. Psoriasis
d. Sarcoidosis
e. Diabetes

14 In DCM, the following are commonly found on echo:
a. Delayed MV closure
b. Decreased mitral E-point to septal separation on M-mode
c. ASD
d. Dilated atria
e. None of the above

15 The following are recognised causes of non-ischaemic DCM:
a. Viral infection
b. Hypertension
c. Alcohol
d. Drugs
e. Peripartum

16 The following are recognised echo findings in ischaemic heart disease:
a. Regional wall motion abnormalities
b. Apical VSD in anterior MI
c. LV aneurysms
d. MR in posterior MI
e. All of the above

17 The following are true of RWMA:
a. MIs are the commonest cause
b. Can lead to errors in ejection fraction calculations using M-mode

   c. Sarcoidosis is a recognised cause

   d. When discovered, tissue Doppler techniques can be useful is assessing LV function

   e. Hypereosinophilic syndrome is a recognised cause

18 With regard to ischaemic heart disease, the following are true:

   a. Finding akinetic myocardium always means irreversible damage has occurred

   b. Circumflex artery occlusion can produce a lateral wall motion defect

   c. LV thrombus is frequently found even when LV function is preserved

   d. It may lead to ventricular dyssynchrony

   e. The right coronary artery cannot be seen on TTE

19 The following are true of LV aneurysms:

   a. False aneurysms are rarely lined with thrombus

   b. True aneurysms have a narrow neck

   c. True aneurysms are lined by thinned myocardium

   d. Can be caused by Chagas' disease

   e. Infero-basal aneurysms are the most common type

20 The following are true of hypertrophic cardiomyopathy:

   a. Systolic dysfunction is common

   b. Certain treatments of LVOT obstruction can lead to RWMA

   c. May be localised entirely to the apex

   d. Can cause MR

   e. Fabry's disease can give a similar echocardiographic appearance

21 The following are recognised causes of biatrial enlargement on echocardiography:

   a. Amyloidosis

   b. Atrial fibrillation

   c. Persistent left sided SVC

   d. Aortic dissection

   e. Isolated left ventricular non-compaction

22 The following favour RCM over DCM:

   a. Preserved systolic function

   b. Biatrial enlargement

    c. dP/dT of >1000
    d. Paradoxical septal motion
    e. Small ventricles

23 The following are associated with HOCM:
    a. Asymmetrical septal hypertrophy
    b. VSD
    c. Early closure of the aortic valve
    d. Peak aortic velocity on CW Doppler at the end of systole
    e. Exhibits dynamic outflow tract obstruction that varies with preload and afterload

24 The following are true of DCM:
    a. Is easily distinguishable from end-stage ischaemic cardiomyopathy
    b. Can be echocardiographically indistinguishable from end-stage RCM
    c. Is a substrate for LV thrombus formation
    d. Respiratory variation across tricuspid valve Doppler flow should always be measured
    e. Often causes AR

25 The following are true regarding severe LV systolic impairment:
    a. Can cause spontaneous echo contrast
    b. Ridging of the endocardium on colour flow is seen in association with isolated LV non-compaction
    c. Is commonly seen in Fabry's disease
    d. May underestimate the severity of AS
    e. The dP/dT ratio is reduced

26 Regarding normal LV function:
    a. The early diastolic filling phase is due to atrial contraction
    b. The IVCT is different from IVRT in that the valves are not closed in the former
    c. The IVCT is not required for calculation of the myocardial performance index
    d. There is both transverse and longitudinal contraction
    e. Systolic velocity is away from the transducer in tissue Doppler in the apical 4-chamber view

27 In a completely normal heart:
    a. Stroke volume is equal in all chambers
    b. The RV and LV should measure the same size in the apical 4-chamber view
    c. The TV is closer to the apex than the MV
    d. A D-shaped LV is commonly seen in the parasternal short-axis view
    e. The LVEDD is usually <5.9 cm in men

28 The following are true of normal cardiac anatomy:
    a. A prominent septal bulge can be seen in elderly people
    b. Atrial septal aneurysms are an incidental finding
    c. A PA diameter in the parasternal short-axis view of 2.7 cm is normal
    d. Persistent left-sided SVC drainage into the coronary sinus is seen in otherwise normal hearts
    e. Flow is laminar in unobstructed vessels

29 With reference to the left ventricular IVRT:
    a. It can vary with heart rate
    b. Refers to the time when there is a fall in pressure but not volume change in the LV
    c. Can be normal or decreased in diastolic dysfunction
    d. The left-sided valves are always closed
    e. Can be measured using PW Doppler

30 The following are true regarding quantitative assessment of LV function:
    a. The Simpson's rule uses a summation of discs from apex to base
    b. Teichholz method of LV function assessment is superior to Simpson's method
    c. In the single plane ellipsoid method, the single plane used is a short-axis view.
    d. Accurate assessment depends on good endocardial border definition
    e. In the Simpson's biplane method, the apical 2- and 4-chamber views are used

Left Ventricular Assessment

ANSWERS

1 a. T
  b. T
  c. T
  d. F
  e. F

Fabry's disease may produce a binary appearance of the LV endocardial border due to compartmentalisation of glycosphingolipids. Amyloidosis leads to a characteristic speckling of the myocardium. Systolic anterior motion of the mitral valve in hypertrophic cardiomyopathy is also well recognised. However, myocarditis tends to produce global LV impairment (RWMA are sometimes seen) whereas Tako–Tsubo cardiomyopathy produces transient apical ballooning.

2 a. F
  b. T
  c. F
  d. T
  e. T

LVH is not an acute process; acute infarction will in any case cause regional wall dysfunction and myocardial thinning. Dilated cardiomyopathies are also generally associated with thinning of the myocardial walls. HCM is a recognised cause of asymmetrical LVH and hypertension leads to concentric, symmetrical LVH. RCM is often due to infiltration of the myocardium leading to thickened and stiffened ventricles.

3 a. T
  b. T
  c. F
  d. T
  e. F

Diastolic dysfunction shows an echocardiographic spectrum ranging from impaired ventricular relaxation initially to reduced LV compliance in its advanced stages. E:E' <5 indicates normal function.

4 a. T
  b. F
  c. T
  d. T
  e. F

Mild–moderate diastolic dysfunction is associated with impaired LV relaxation, which causes a prolonged deceleration time in transmitral flow and E:A ratio reversal. The IVRT is usually prolonged, but normalises when LA pressures become elevated in moderate disease. The pulmonary vein flow readings suggest severe diastolic dysfunction.

5 a. T
  b. T
  c. T
  d. T
  e. F

There is normally a slight variation in transmitral and tricuspid flow with breathing; this is exaggerated in tamponade leading to pulsus paradoxus. Both preload (e.g. IV fluid overload) and afterload (aortic resistance) affect systolic function. Normal cardiac output is around 5 l/min in men and 4 l/min in women. It can rise to 15–20 l/min during exercise. Isovolumic contraction is short in normal systolic function with a rapid rise to peak pressure; both are altered with impaired function.

6 a. T
  b. T
  c. F
  d. T
  e. T

Stiffness is the inverse of compliance. Myocardial relaxation is an active (energy-requiring) process. LA filling may transiently fall in inspiration as blood 'pools' in the pulmonary vasculature due to increased negative intra-thoracic pressures; LA filling is maximal therefore in end-expiration. In severe diastolic dysfunction, the LV is often stiff and non-compliant, therefore most LV filling occurs early in diastole causing a large transmitral E wave and comparatively smaller A wave.

7 a. T
   b. T
   c. F
   d. T
   e. F

The presence of pericardial calcification and constrictive physiology would restrict the ability of the LV to fully distend and therefore fill properly. Atrial fibrillation reduces diastolic LV filling through loss of the transmitral A wave and dehydration through simple loss of vascular volume. Bradycardia increases diastolic time and hence increases filling. MR causes increased transmitral flow and eventually elevated LA pressures, both increasing diastolic filling of the LV.

8 a. T
   b. F
   c. F
   d. F
   e. T

dP/dT is calculated by applying the Bernoulli equation i.e. $4(V_2^2 - V_1^2) \div dT$. Thus, $4(3)^2 - 4(1)^2 \div 0.04 = 32 \div 0.04 = 800$ (normal range >1000 mmHg/s). Fractional shortening is [(LVEDD − LVESD) ÷ LVEDD] × 100%. Thus, [(6.3 − 4.9) ÷ 6.3] × 100 = 22% (normal range 25–45%).

Clearly, LV function is impaired. The patient has likely had a RCA or possibly Circumflex territory infarct. MR is a recognised complication of posterior infarcts.

9 a. T
   b. T
   c. T
   d. F
   e. T

The key calculation is the SV. SV = Area$(\pi r^2)_{LVOT}$ × VTI$_{LVOT}$. Thus, SV = $\pi(1.4)^2$ × 8 = 49 ml.
EF = [SV ÷ LVED volume] × 100. Therefore, LVED volume = 100 SV ÷ EF = 4900 ÷ 50 = 100 ml.
Cardiac output = SV × HR. Cardiac output = 49 × 90 = 4.4 l/min

The antero-apical region is subtended by the LAD coronary artery; the patient has therefore had an anterior infarct and does not have AS. Apical VSDs are a complication of anterior MIs.

10 a. F
  b. T
  c. T
  d. F
  e. T

LV midwall fibres are orientated circumferentially, whereas subendocardial and subepicardial fibres are longitudinal. Tissue Doppler imaging reveals that short-axis function is generally preserved with age whereas long-axis function does deteriorate. It also shows that the endocardium moves faster than the epicardium. If severe MR is present, colour M-mode should produce a near vertical slope with normal LV function and systolic PV flow is normally slightly higher than diastolic flow.

11 a. F
  b. T
  c. T
  d. F
  e. F

LVH is only mild–moderate and the LA with a volume of 60 ml is mildly dilated under current BSE guidance (normal range 22–52 ml for women). Although the IVRT is normal, there is LVH and the LA is dilated in a patient with symptoms so the patient has diastolic dysfunction. The normal IVRT suggests that this is moderate dysfunction and the E:A ratio is pseudonormalised. Tissue Doppler E/E′ <5 is in keeping with normal diastolic function. A deceleration time of < 100 ms suggests severe diastolic impairment.

12 a. T
  b. F
  c. F
  d. T
  e. T

Concentric and symmetrical thickening of >2 cm is consistent with severe LVH. The step-up in mid-cavity gradient is due to late systolic obliteration but the diagnosis here is hypertensive cardiomyopathy, rather than primary hypertrophic obstructive cardiomyopathy. There is no severe AV disease that requires surgery and an aortic root of 4 cm does not require replacement The AR jet represents the gradient between the aorta and LVOT. By applying the Bernoulli equation, this is $4(4.2)^2 = 71$ mmHg. Subtracting this from the diastolic BP gives the LVEDP $= 100 - 71 = 29$ mmHg

13 a. T
   b. T
   c. F
   d. T
   e. F

The main causes of restrictive cardiomyopathies are infiltrative processes such as amyloid, haemochromatosis or glycogen storage diseases. Multisystem inflammatory disorders such as sarcoidosis and the hypereosinophilic syndrome are also causes. Psoriasis can cause high-output cardiac failure similar to thyrotoxicosis, but diabetes does not cause an infiltrative cardiomyopathy; it is associated with heart failure with normal ejection fraction and coronary artery disease.

14 a. T
   b. F
   c. F
   d. T
   e. F

M-mode through the LV in parasternal long axis shows the delayed MV closure in DCM as a 'B-bump' due to an elevated LVEDP. The E-point septal separation represents the distance between the septum and the MV leaflet during its E-wave phase – this distance is increased in DCM, which is a dilatation of all four chambers, including both atria. However, ASDs are not usually found.

15 a. T
   b. F
   c. T
   d. T
   e. T

There are a number of causes of non-ischaemic DCM, but viral infections, drugs (e.g. anthracyclines) and alcohol are the most common. Peripartum cardiomyopathy is also recognised, presenting most often in the month before delivery. Hypertension generally causes concentric LVH.

16 a. T
  b. T
  c. T
  d. T
  e. T
All are true.

17 a. T
  b. T
  c. T
  d. T
  e. F
Ischaemic heart disease is the commonest cause of RWMAs. When present, standard M-mode measurements of basal LV dimensions for ejection fraction will not account for loss of apical function; Simpson's method should be used in this setting. Tissue Doppler can assess regional wall function. Sarcoidosis can cause regional wall motion defects and conduction disturbances, whereas the hypereosinophilic syndrome is a rare cause of LV thrombus in the absence of regional wall motion defects.

18 a. F
  b. T
  c. F
  d. T
  e. F
In acute ischaemia, akinetic myocardium may indicate stunned or hibernating myocardium that may regain normal contractile function if revascularisation occurs early. The circumflex artery supplies the lateral and sometimes the posterior wall. In ischaemia, LV thrombus is almost always found in the context of reduced LV function. Dyssynchrony can result from damage to the bundle branch conduction pathways. The RCA can be seen in the parasternal short-axis view.

19 a. F
  b. F
  c. T
  d. T
  e. F
False aneurysms have a narrow neck and thrombus is a characteristic feature; true aneurysms have a wide neck, tapered edge and the

involved myocardium is usually thinned. Chagas' disease can cause aneurysms and is exceptional in that it has almost no involvement of the ventricular septum. Apical aneurysms are by far the commonest type.

20 a. F
  b. T
  c. T
  d. T
  e. T

Diastolic dysfunction is common in HCM, while systolic function is generally preserved until a late stage. HCM with drug-refractory dynamic outflow obstruction can be treated with alcohol septal ablation. This essentially causes an infarction of the ventricular septum causing a regional defect. Although there are variations in echocardiographic appearance, apical HCM is well recognised. MR can result from systolic anterior motion of the MV leaflet. Fabry's disease (an x-linked lysozomal storage disorder) causes ventricular hypertrophy and septal thickening similar to HCM.

21 a. T
  b. T
  c. F
  d. F
  e. F

Amyloid and most forms of the restrictive cardiomyopathies will cause biatrial enlargement. Longstanding atrial fibrillation can also cause this. A persistent left-sided SVC may cause a dilated coronary sinus and possibly right atrial but not biatrial enlargement. Similarly, aortic dissection may cause a dilated aortic root, but not biatrial enlargement. Isolated left ventricular non-compaction causes deep inter-trabecular recesses in the ventricular myocardium and has no direct effect on the atria.

22 a. T
  b. F
  c. T
  d. F
  e. T

Systolic function is usually preserved in RCM but impaired in DCM. Biatrial enlargement occurs in both and is not discriminatory. dP/dT >1000 suggests normal systolic function and does not favour

DCM. Paradoxical septal motion suggests RV volume overload or dyskinesia from bundle branch block, neither of which distinguish RCM from DCM. Although biatrial enlargement occurs in both cardiomyopathies, RCM is associated with small ventricles whereas DCM has dilated ventricles.

23 a. T
   b. F
   c. T
   d. T
   e. T

Asymmetrical septal hypertrophy is commonly seen in HCM with and without obstruction. VSDs are not a recognised association. Patients with dynamic outflow tract obstruction exhibit mid-systolic aortic valve closure. Peak aortic velocity is seen at end-systole as this is when the LVOT (or mid-cavity/apex) is at its narrowest, creating the highest velocity. Outflow tract obstruction is dependent on many factors, such as hydration, heart rate, squatting, etc.

24 a. F
   b. T
   c. T
   d. F
   e. F

End-stage ischaemic cardiomyopathy causes wall thinning and global reduction in systolic function similar to DCM. The same is true of end-stage RCM. Poor LV function is common in DCM, and this predisposes to thrombus formation. Respiratory variation across the TV is useful in suspected tamponade and plays little part in the assessment of DCM. Dilatation of the aortic root causing AR is not commonly seen; indeed concomitant AR would suggest primary valve pathology.

25 a. T
   b. T
   c. F
   d. T
   e. T

Severe LV impairment causes sluggish blood flow, which is thought to be related to the appearance of spontaneous echo contrast. Isolated LV non-compaction is uncommon and produces severe LV dysfunction with deep trabecular recesses, manifest as ridging on echo. Systolic function is generally preserved in Fabry's disease. Systolic impairment may underestimate the severity of AS if the Bernoulli equation is used; it is better to calculate the valve area in this instance to grade severity. dP/dT ratio in the transmitral regurgitant jet is a marker of systolic function, and is therefore reduced.

26 a. F
   b. F
   c. F
   d. T
   e. F

It is the late diastolic filling phase that is due to atrial contraction, the early filling phase is passive due to opening of the MV. Both the MV and AV are closed during both IVCT and IVRT, hence there is no movement of blood (isovolumic). Myocardial perfusion index is the (IVCT + IVRT) ÷ ejection time. The normal arrangement of myocardial fibres is such that there is both transverse and longitudinal contraction. Normal systolic velocities are towards the transducer in tissue Doppler in the apical 4-chamber view whereas diastolic velocities are away.

27 a. T
   b. F
   c. T
   d. F
   e. T

In a completely normal heart, SV is the same in each chamber. The LV is larger and thicker walled than the RV and the TV is more apically displaced than the MV. Finding a D-shaped LV on parasternal short axis is a pathological finding, suggesting the presence of pulmonary hypertension and/or RV overload. The LVED dimension is usually less than 6 cm.

28 a. T
   b. T
   c. F
   d. T
   e. T

A septal prominence close to the LVOT is common in elderly people and must not be mistaken for HCM. Atrial septal aneurysms can be seen in all age groups and are often a coincidental finding. In the parasternal short-axis view, a PA diameter of up to 2.2 cm would be considered normal; 2.7 cm would be moderately dilated. Left-sided SVC drainage into the coronary sinus is occasionally seen in routine echocardiograms of young patients as an apparent cystic cavity in the LA. Injection of agitated saline into the left arm veins delineates the true nature. Flow in unobstructed vessels is laminar whereas flow through a stenosis causes disordered non-uniform flow.

29 a. T
   b. T
   c. T
   d. T
   e. T

The IVRT does vary with heart rate and represents the time when the LV is relaxing, which lowers the ventricular pressure. Assuming a BP of 120/80, then peak LV pressure is 120 mmHg; as the pressure drops to approximately 80 mmHg, the AV will close. As the MV will not open until LV pressure continues to drop to about 5–10 mmHg, all left-sided valves are closed for the duration of the IVRT and there can be no volume change. In moderate–severe diastolic dysfunction, the IVRT is either normal or decreased and it can be measured by placing a PW Doppler midway between the MV and AV in the apical 5-chamber view, so that transmitral and transaortic flows are picked up; the time duration between them is the IVRT.

30 a. T
   b. F
   c. F
   d. T
   e. T

2D echo is a tomographic technique and assumptions regarding the shape of the LV e.g. cylindrical, elliptical, etc. are the basis of these calculations. The Simpson's Rule uses an apical biplane method of assessing LV volumes and essentially splits the LV into (usually) 20 discs; the apical 2- and 4-chamber views are used. The single-plane ellipsoid method uses a single long-axis view. Clearly, the better the endocardial border definition, the more accurate the measurement.

4 The Mitral Valve

QUESTIONS

For each question below, decide whether the answers provided are true or false.

1 The normal MV:
   a. Is made up of two leaflets each with three lobes or scallops
   b. Is in continuity with the AV, via the anterior leaflet
   c. Is more apically positioned than the TV
   d. Is the most posterior valve seen in the parasternal long-axis view
   e. Is attached to the papillary muscles by the chordae tendinae

2 The following are recognised causes of mitral regurgitation:
   a. Infective endocarditis
   b. MI
   c. Myxomatous leaflets
   d. Rheumatic disease
   e. LV dilatation

3 In the parasternal views:
   a. PISA can be optimally imaged and measured
   b. The direction of the regurgitant jet can be identified
   c. E and A waves can be measured
   d. Measurement of the degree of MVP in the parasternal long-axis view is less accurate than that in apical 4-chamber view
   e. The presence of mitral annular calcification can be identified

Successful Accreditation in Echocardiography: A Self-Assessment Guide,
First Edition. Sanjay M. Banypersad and Keith Pearce.
© 2012 John Wiley & Sons, Ltd. Published 2012 by John Wiley & Sons, Ltd.

4 The following are true of MR:
  a. The apical 4-chamber and parasternal long-axis views give the best qualitative assessment of severity
  b. The LA usually dilates with chronic MR
  c. Posterior leaflet prolapse causes a posterior jet of regurgitation.
  d. EF increases in acute MR
  e. A broad-based jet is a marker of severity

5 When assessing MR, the following are true regarding vena contracta:
  a. Vena contracta refers to the narrowest diameter of the regurgitant jet
  b. May be used if an eccentric jet is seen
  c. Is largely independent of flow rate and LV pressures
  d. Is best assessed in the apical 2-chamber view
  e. If >0.7 cm suggests severe MR

6 A 64-year-old man has an echo for increasing breathlessness. The apical 4-chamber view reveals MR on colour flow. A proximal isovelocity surface area with a radius of 1.1 cm is seen with an aliasing velocity of 35 cm/s. The CW Doppler of the MR jet shows a peak velocity of 4.2 m/s and VTI_{MR} of 150 cm. The following are true:
  a. PISA = $7.6 \, cm^2$
  b. Maximum instantaneous regurgitant flow is 190 ml/sec
  c. Maximum instantaneous orifice area is $0.63 \, cm^2$
  d. Actual regurgitant volume over systole is 55–60 ml.
  e. The CW signal for the MR would be expected to be as dense as antegrade flow.

7 The following suggest severe rather than moderate MR:
  a. Regurgitant volume of 50 ml per beat
  b. Regurgitant orifice area of $0.5 \, cm^2$
  c. Pulmonary vein systolic flow reversal
  d. An eccentric jet
  e. Low-density CW signal with a peak velocity of >4 m/s

8 The following echo findings are recognised complications of severe MR:
  a. Systolic anterior motion of the MV
  b. Pulmonary hypertension

   c. An absent A wave on PW Doppler

   d. Slow rise to peak velocity of the regurgitant jet on CW Doppler

   e. RWMA

9 The following are true of MR:
   a. PV systolic flow reversal may not be seen in severe MR if the LA is very dilated
   b. A regurgitant fraction of 25% suggests moderate MR
   c. Is unique in that it is not subject to the choanda effect
   d. A regurgitant jet of 50% LA area suggests moderate MR
   e. Prominent E waves on transmitral flow may be seen

10 The following are true regarding abnormalities of the MV:
   a. Perforation of the valve leaflets implies an ischaemic aetiology
   b. An abnormal posterior leaflet would be best seen in the apical 2-chamber view
   c. Marfan's syndrome is associated with a long, redundant anterior leaflet
   d. A cleft MV can look similar to the TV
   e. MVP always causes MR

11 MS:
   a. Is most commonly caused by rheumatic fever
   b. Does not cause LA dilatation as in MR
   c. Causes fusion of the anterior and posterior leaflets along medial and lateral commissures
   d. Shows doming of the valve leaflets
   e. With a valve area of $1.7\,cm^2$ would be considered severe

12 The following are true regarding assessment of MS by the pressure half-time method:
   a. May underestimate MS with coexisting aortic regurgitation
   b. May overestimate MS with coexisting aortic regurgitation
   c. A pressure half time of 175 ms indicates severe stenosis
   d. Accuracy is dependent on the intercept angle of the probe
   e. Is accurate within 24 h after balloon valvuloplasty

13 The following are true of MS:
   a. The continuity equation requires a coexisting regurgitant jet to be present to calculate MV area.

b. The deceleration slope should be linear when using the pressure half-time method

c. Rheumatic heart disease causes aortic stenosis more commonly than MS

d. Thrombus in the LA may be seen even in sinus rhythm

e. A low Wilkins' score suggests valve replacement should be considered over valvuloplasty

14 When using planimetry for calculating the orifice area in MS:

a. The apical 4-chamber is the optimal view

b. Overestimation of the valve area can result from the gains being too high

c. Underestimation of the valve area may result from measuring too close to the LA

d. Compares well with valve areas calculated with cardiac catheter data

e. This method is more accurate than pressure half time when image quality is poor

15 The following are true of MS:

a. Doppler assessment is independent of HR

b. Severe aortic regurgitation can produce functional MS even when the MV is normal

c. The presence of an ASD would invalidate the pressure half-time method

d. MR can result from balloon valvuloplasty

e. An ASD can result from balloon valvuloplasty

16 The following are markers of severity in MS:

a. Valve area $<1\,cm^2$

b. Pressure gradient $>15\,mmHg$

c. AF

d. The presence of leaflet thickening

e. Decreased E–F slope

17 You perform an echo on a young Sudanese woman with MS. CW Doppler shows a transmitral VTI of 78 cm and an E:A ratio of 1. The PA diameter is 2 cm with a transpulmonary VTI of 20 cm. There is no regurgitation seen, except for physiological TR with a peak velocity of 3.5 m/s. The following are true:

a. Planimetry of the mitral valve orifice in short axis would be expected to yield an area of approximately $0.8\,cm^2$

b. The pressure half time would be expected to be 275 ms
c. Pulmonary hypertension is present
d. Atrial fibrillation is present
e. The transmitral pressure gradient cannot be calculated from the data given

18 In MS:
a. M-mode may show anterior movement of the posterior leaflet
b. The Wilkins' score assesses both leaflet thickening and mobility
c. The majority of patients are male
d. Diastolic closure of the MV is later than normal
e. TOE is not necessary prior to balloon valvuloplasty

19 The following are recognised in MVP:
a. Can only be definitively assessed at angiography
b. Both leaflets must billow into the LA by at least 6 mm by definition
c. Prolapse of other valves may be associated
d. Carries a poor prognosis
e. Can be found in association with Marfan's syndrome

20 With regard to the MV
a. Functional MR may be seen with dilated cardiomyopathy
b. The anterior leaflet is the larger leaflet by area
c. The anterior leaflet subtends a larger circumference of the annulus
d. In asymptomatic severe MR due to leaflet prolapse, an end-systolic dimension of >4.5 cm is an indication for surgery
e. In asymptomatic severe MR due to leaflet prolapse, the onset of AF is an indication for surgery

The Mitral Valve

ANSWERS

1 a. T
  b. T
  c. F
  d. T
  e. T

From a nomenclature point of view in echocardiography, the MV is made up of an anterior and posterior leaflet, each divided into three scallops. The anterior leaflet is in fibrous continuity with the AV, but the TV is more apically positioned than the MV; this aids identification of the ventricles in complex congenital heart disease. The chordae tendinae attach the leaflets to the papillary muscle apparatus.

2 a. T
  b. T
  c. T
  d. T
  e. T

All are recognised causes of MR.

3 a. F
  b. T
  c. F
  d. F
  e. T

The 4-chamber view is the optimal view for imaging PISA and for using PW Doppler for E and A wave measurements. The direction of the jet can be assessed in the parasternal long and short axes, as can annular calcification. The annulus of the MV is saddle-shaped and the lowest portion of it is not seen in the apical 4-chamber view, therefore prolapse past the annulus cannot be accurately assessed in this view. The parasternal long axis is a superior view in this regard.

4 a. T
  b. T
  c. F
  d. T
  e. T

The apical 4-chamber and parasternal long-axis views provide good visual assessments with colour Doppler and allow quantitative assessments with CW Doppler too. A dilated LA is often seen in chronic MR whereas in acute MR, the LA may not have had time to dilate and LV volumes are ejected into the LA in addition to the aorta, hence EF will increase. Posterior leaflet prolapse will cause anteriorly directed regurgitation and a broad-based jet indicates severe MR.

5 a. T
  b. T
  c. T
  d. F
  e. T

The vena contracta is the narrowest neck of the regurgitant jet, usually just at the point of entry into the LA. If eccentric jets are seen, it may not be possible to angulate the CW Doppler probe such that it is parallel to the jet, so measurement of the vena contracta is a more accurate marker of severity in this instance. Vena contractae sizes are mainly determined by the orifice area, and are therefore independent of LV function and flow rate. It can be visualised in any of the standard views, although the apical 2-chamber view can show a broad-based jet even though regurgitation is not severe because of the plane of imaging and should not be used. Measurement >0.7 cm suggests severe MR.

6 a. T
  b. F
  c. T
  d. F
  e. T

PISA is $2\pi r^2$, therefore for a radius of 1.1 cm, PISA = 7.6 cm^2. The maximum instantaneous regurgitant flow (RV_{max}) is PISA × aliasing velocity i.e. 7.6 × 35 = 266 ml/s and the corresponding orifice area (ROA) is calculated by $RV_{max} \div V_{MR}$ which is 266 ÷ 4.2 = 0.63 cm^2. *Actual* regurgitant volume over systole is given by ROA × VTI_{MR} which is 0.63 × 150 = 94 cm^3 or 94 ml. These calculations are all in keeping with severe MR and the CW signal therefore would be as dense as forward flow through the MV.

7 a. F
  b. T
  c. T
  d. F
  e. F

A regurgitant volume of 30–60 ml/beat is considered moderate, greater than 60 ml/beat is severe. Pulmonary vein systolic flow reversal is in keeping with severe MR as is ROA of 0.5 cm^2. The direction of the jet may give an indication of aetiology but is not a marker of severity per se. Similarly, peak velocity of the regurgitant jet of >4 m/s alone is not sufficient to indicate severe MR over moderate MR, unless significant PISA was also present or the CW signal was very dense.

8 a. F
  b. T
  c. T
  d. T
  e. F

Systolic anterior motion is a complication of HCM leading to MR, it is not a complication of MR. Pulmonary hypertension is a common complication of chronic severe MR. AF is frequently seen in severe MR, which leads to the absence of the A wave. A slow rise to peak velocity suggests impaired LV function, which may also be a consequence of severe MR and is an indication for valve surgery, as is the development of pulmonary hypertension. RWMAs are not complications of severe MR but may be seen in conjunction with it, such as in posterior MI causing posterior akinesia, ruptured chordae and thus MR.

9 a. T
  b. F
  c. F
  d. F
  e. T

With chronic MR, the LA may become very dilated, when even severe MR may not reach the pulmonary veins. A regurgitant fraction of 30–50% and a jet area of 20–40% both indicate moderate MR. Any regurgitant jet can be subject to the choanda effect if eccentric jets 'adhere' to the LA wall. Prominent E waves may be seen as LA pressures are increased with MR.

10 a. F
b. F
c. T
d. T
e. F

Perforation of the leaflets implies endocarditis as the aetiology. The apical 2-chamber view images primarily the anterior leaflet and abnormalities of the posterior leaflet will therefore not be readily evident. Marfan's syndrome is associated with a long, redundant anterior leaflet as well as MVP and aortic regurgitation. A cleft MV does look anatomically similar to the TV and indeed can be difficult to distinguish from the TV in the presence of congenital heart disease. MVP can be present with and without MR; this is often best visualised in parasternal long-axis or apical 2-chamber views.

11 a. T
b. F
c. T
d. T
e. F

The most common cause is childhood rheumatic fever, followed by calcific disease. MS can cause very dilated left atria and is a substrate for LA thrombus. Commissural fusion is characteristic of MS, and is typically along the medial and lateral commissures. In the parasternal long axis, MS can be seen as doming or bowing of the valve leaflets. A valve area of $1.7\,cm^2$ is in the mild stenosis category.

12 a. T
b. T
c. F
d. T
e. F

The pressure half-time method has a number of limitations. Coexisting aortic regurgitation means LV diastolic pressures rise more rapidly causing the pressure half time to be shortened, which overestimates the orifice area and thus underestimates the true stenosis. An eccentric jet of AR restricts the opening of the anterior mitral leaflet in diastole, causing functional MS in addition to the existing stenosis, which would prolong the pressure half time, underestimating the orifice area and therefore overestimating the true degree of stenosis. A time of 175 ms represents moderate MS. The position of the probe is crucial for accurate assessment by Doppler and must be parallel to the regurgitant jet. Immediately after valvuloplasty, chamber compliances between the LA and LV take up to 72 h to reach equilibrium, so the pressure half-time method is not accurate in this setting.

13 a. F
  b. T
  c. F
  d. T
  e. F

The continuity equation only requires that SV be known and the VTI of the stenotic jet. The presence of a regurgitant jet is not required and indeed may invalidate the calculation. When using the pressure half-time method, the deceleration slope should ideally be linear though this is not always attainable. The MV is more commonly affected than the AV in rheumatic heart disease. MS can cause left atrial thrombus to develop even in sinus rhythm as obstruction to blood flow out of the LA causes blood to stagnate; consequently, whereas patients with MR and dilated LA are often commenced on warfarin therapy when in atrial fibrillation, patients with MS are often commenced on warfarin even in sinus rhythm. A low Wilkins' score suggests a good candidate for valve commissurotomy (or valvuloplasty), not valve replacement.

14 a. F
  b. F
  c. F
  d. T
  e. F

The optimal view is the parasternal short axis, facing the valve head-on. One should scan from the apex to the first point that the MV tips appear, this is the narrowest part of the valve orifice. Tracing round the orifice higher up (closer to the LA) will inevitably overestimate the valve area. If the gains are too high, the valve will appear to be thicker than it is, with the luminal edges seemingly encroaching into the orifice; planimetry may thus cause the valve area to be underestimated. Planimetry has been well validated against cardiac catheter data, but is not accurate when image quality is poor, as visualisation of the orifice is suboptimal.

15 a. F
   b. T
   c. T
   d. T
   e. T

Using Doppler to assess valve area is dependent on HR because at high HRs, LA filling per beat is reduced as the cardiac cycle is shorter and transmitral flow terminates earlier as diastole is shorter. Severe AR, especially if posteriorly directed, can impinge on the anterior leaflet of the MV, restricting its opening causing functional MS. ASDs invalidate the pressure half-time method as blood will shunt from the LA across to the RA. During balloon valvuloplasty, the LA is accessed via a trans-septal puncture from the RA, which can leave an ASD. As the stenotic valve is then dilated with the balloon, the leaflets can be torn leading to a regurgitant valve.

16 a. T
   b. T
   c. F
   d. F
   e. F

Markers of severity in MS are a valve area of $<1 \, cm^2$ and a gradient of $>15 \, mmHg$. AF is a complication of MS but is not a marker of severity. Coexisting leaflet thickening may be suggestive of aetiology but is not a marker of severity. A decreased E–F slope is seen on M-mode across the MV in MS but again does not correlate well with severity as it is affected by annular motion and fibrosis among other factors.

17 a. T
   b. T
   c. T
   d. F
   e. T

The valve area can be calculated using the continuity equation, such that: Valve $Area_{PULM} \times VTI_{PULM} =$ Valve $Area_{MITRAL} \times VTI_{MITRAL}$. Therefore, mitral valve area $= [[\pi(1)^2 \times 20]] \div] \, 78 = 0.8 \, cm^2$. Knowing that MV area is also equal to $220 \div$ pressure half time, it is clear that the pressure half time is $275 \, ms$. The pulmonary pressure is calculated from the TR jet velocity using the Bernoulli equation i.e. $4v^2 = 4(3.5)^2 = 49$ mmHg. Atrial fibrillation is not present because the A wave is seen on CW Doppler. The pressure gradient cannot be calculated from the data given, as the peak velocity of the stenotic jet is not known.

18 a. T
   b. T
   c. F
   d. T
   e. F

Normal MV leaflets move in opposite directions in diastole, but in MS, the posterior leaflet moves upwards with the anterior leaflet on M-mode. The Wilkins' score assesses leaflet thickening, mobility, calcification and the subvalvular apparatus. The majority of MS patients are female. Diastolic closure of the MV is later than normal in MS because the persistent gradient from LA to LV in diastole keeps the valve open for longer. TOE is mandatory prior to valvuloplasty as it has a higher sensitivity and specificity for detecting thrombus in the left atrial appendage than TTE.

19 a. F
   b. F
   c. T
   d. F
   e. T

Angiography is never required to diagnose MVP. Part of one or both leaflets must rise above the mitral annulus (in the parasternal long-axis or apical 3-chamber views) by at least 2 mm for the diagnosis. Prolapse of the TV and AV is seen in approximately 20% patients with MVP. Isolated MVP carries an excellent prognosis, and such patients should have follow-up scans every 3–5 years. MVP is associated with other conditions, such as Marfan's syndrome, Ehlers–Danlos syndrome and osteogenesis imperfecta.

20 a. T
   b. T
   c. F
   d. T
   e. T

Dilatation of the LV cavity leads to stretching of the mitral annulus and non-coaptation of the valve leaflets, leading to a central jet known as functional MR. The anterior leaflet is the larger leaflet by area but it is the posterior leaflet that subtends the larger annular circumference of the two. In severe, asymptomatic MR, the indications for surgery under current European (ESC) guidance are LV dilatation (end-systolic >4.5 cm), LV dysfunction, AF or pulmonary hypertension. The American (ACC/AHA) guidelines differ slightly in that surgery is considered when the end-systolic dimensions reach 4 cm.

5 Right Ventricular Assessment

QUESTIONS

For each question below, decide whether the answers provided are true or false.

1 With regard to the anatomy of the RV:
   a. Chamber size is normally the same as the LV
   b. Wall thickness is normally the same as the LV
   c. The body of the RV is anterior to the LV
   d. In the parasternal long-axis inflow view, septal and posterior leaflets of the TV are seen
   e. In the parasternal long-axis inflow view, the diameter of the RV should be measured at a point ⅓ of the way into the RV from the tricuspid annulus

2 The following are recognised causes of pulmonary arterial hypertension:
   a. Ischaemic cardiomyopathy with LV dysfunction
   b. MR
   c. Connective tissue disease
   d. Pulmonary embolic disease
   e. Left to right shunts

3 The following are causes of RVH:
   a. TR
   b. Arrhythmogenic right ventricular cardiomyopathy
   c. PS
   d. Aortic dissection
   e. Congenitally corrected transposition of the great vessels

Successful Accreditation in Echocardiography: A Self-Assessment Guide,
First Edition. Sanjay M. Banypersad and Keith Pearce.
© 2012 John Wiley & Sons, Ltd. Published 2012 by John Wiley & Sons, Ltd.

4 The following are true of the TV:
   a. Is preferentially affected by carcinoid disease compared with the MV
   b. Abnormalities of the TV are the commonest cardiac defect in Down syndrome
   c. Is harvested as part of the Ross procedure
   d. Is at a higher risk of endocarditis in IV drug abusers compared with left-sided valves
   e. Is normally located 0.5–1 cm more apically than the MV

5 The following are true regarding right heart valvular disease:
   a. Severe TR causes systolic flow reversal in the vena cava
   b. Trivial–mild PR may be considered normal
   c. The PR jet velocity can be used to calculate diastolic PA pressure
   d. A TR jet velocity of 4.5 m/s indicates severe TR
   e. In pulmonary hypertension, directly measuring peak systolic PA velocity to assess PA pressure is more accurate than calculating it from the TR jet velocity

6 PS is commonly seen in association with:
   a. Noonan's syndrome
   b. Arrhythmogenic right ventricular cardiomyopathy
   c. Tetralogy of Fallot
   d. Transposition of the great vessels
   e. Alagille's syndrome

7 The following statements can be considered true when assessing the RV:
   a. An RV systolic area >15 cm^2 is abnormal
   b. An RV diastolic area >25 cm^2 would be considered abnormal
   c. In the parasternal short-axis view, an RVOT diameter of 2 cm at PV level would be normal
   d. In the apical 4-chamber view, a mid-RV diameter of 3.5 cm is mildly dilated
   e. TAPSE >15 mm would be considered normal

8 The following are true of septal motion with abnormalities of the RV:
   a. D-shaped septum in diastole with normal septal movement in systole suggests isolated RV volume overload
   b. D-shaped septum in diastole and systole suggests volume overload with a pressure-overload component
   c. RBBB causes rapid downward septal motion on M-mode

d. Right ventricular dilatation with a flat septum throughout the cardiac cycle implies RV and LV mass is equal

e. RV and RA dilatation with paradoxical septal motion should prompt a search for a defect in the atrial septum

9 The following are true regarding dimensions and Doppler of the right heart:

a. RV wall thickness of >0.5 cm would be considered abnormal

b. An RV end-diastolic diameter of >4 cm in the apical 4-chamber view would be considered abnormal

c. A time to peak velocity of <80 ms in the PA suggests the presence of pulmonary hypertension

d. A PA diameter of 3.5 cm suggests the presence of pulmonary hypertension

e. A shortened right ventricular IVRT is in keeping with pulmonary hypertension

10 You are asked to perform an echo on an 18-year-old female presenting with sudden chest pain and breathlessness. There is moderate TR with a velocity of 3.8 m/s. There is moderate PR with an end-diastolic peak velocity of 3 m/s. The RV is dilated and impaired. The LV is of normal size and appears mildly impaired. The IVC is dilated with <50% collapse on inspiration. The following statements are true:

a. The likely diagnosis is an acute MI

b. Diastolic PA pressure is approximately 36 mmHg

c. Systolic PA pressure is approximately 50 mmHg.

d. Septal motion would be expected to appear normal

e. Thrombolysis should be considered

11 You are called to perform an echo on a 60-year-old man in A&E. His BP is 90/50. A limited study reveals a muscular VSD with left to right flow. The CW Doppler shows this velocity to be 3 m/s. The RV is dilated and the septum is D-shaped in diastole and flat in systole. All valves are functioning normally with no stenosis or regurgitation. The IVC is of normal size and only minimally collapses on inspiration. The following are true:

a. Systolic PA pressure is approximately 50–55 mmHg

b. Systolic PA pressure is approximately 70–75 mmHg

c. Eisenmenger's syndrome is present

d. The pattern of septal motion is due to volume overload alone

e. These findings should prompt a search for a coexistent ASD

12 The following are true regarding anatomy of the right heart:
   a. The moderator band is a prominent muscular band traversing the RV apex
   b. The MV does not have papillary muscle attachments
   c. The IVC enters the RA inferiorly to the coronary sinus
   d. The Chiari network is essentially an extension of the Eustachian valve
   e. The crista terminalis takes a posterior course from the SVC to the IVC

13 The following are true:
   a. Chiari network is associated with ASDs and PFOs
   b. Lushka's muscle is exclusively found in the right heart
   c. Estimated PA pressure calculated from the TR jet may be underestimated in the presence of PS
   d. Respiratory variation of the IVC is not affected in ICU patients who are intubated and ventilated
   e. Time to peak velocity of the PA Doppler signal may appear normal in the co-presence of pulmonary hypertension and RV dysfunction

14 The following are true of assessment of RV function:
   a. EF is around 45% normally
   b. TAPSE is assessed using M-mode
   c. RV function cannot be assessed using Doppler
   d. TAPSE of <1.5 cm is suggestive of RV dysfunction
   e. The Tei index takes into account the intra-ventricular contraction and relaxation times

15 The following are true when assessing the RV:
   a. Localised aneurysms of the RV are in keeping with arrhythmogenic right ventricular cardiomyopathy
   b. Tissue Doppler can identify the isovolumic contraction velocity
   c. Strain rate imaging assesses regional RV function more accurately than tissue Doppler because it measures deformation rather than velocity
   d. A Tei index of >0.4 indicates normal RV function
   e. McConell's sign may be seen in acute PE

16 The following statements are true:
   a. A large increase in tricuspid VTI in inspiration would be in keeping with tamponade
   b. RWMAs of the RV are most commonly due to ARVC

c. An IVC that does not collapse with respiration suggests an RA pressure of around 10 mmHg

d. Elevated right heart pressures may mask features of tamponade

e. The Gerbode defect usually involves a shunt between the RV and the LA

17 The following suggest significant pulmonary hypertension:
   a. Mid-systolic closure of the PV
   b. PR end-diastolic jet velocity of 1.5 m/s
   c. Mid-systolic notch on PA Doppler
   d. Severe TR
   e. Peak PA systolic velocity of 4 m/s

18 The following statements is true when assessing right heart dysfunction:
   a. In the 4-chamber view, a base to apex measurement of 7.5 cm suggests severe RV dilatation
   b. A PISA radius of 0.5 cm suggests severe TR
   c. Dilated hepatic veins suggests an estimated RA pressure of 15–20 mmHg
   d. A regurgitant fraction of 65% suggests moderate PR
   e. In the 4-chamber view, basal RV diameter of 4.5 cm is mildly dilated

19 The following statements are true regarding abnormalities of the right heart:
   a. ARVC only affects the RV
   b. Restrictive cardiomyopathies do not affect the RV
   c. RBBB can produce septal dyssynchrony
   d. The TV is normally more apically positioned compared with the MV
   e. The finding of a ventricular pacing wire against the RVOT septum always suggests displacement from the RV apex position

20 The following are true:
   a. A tricuspid annular velocity of >10 cm/s is normal
   b. The Simpson's biplane method is most appropriate when assessing RV function
   c. Myxomas do not occur in the right heart
   d. Right atrial area by planimetry is usually <20 cm^2
   e. Tricuspid stenosis is rare

Right Ventricular Assessment

ANSWERS

1 a. F
  b. F
  c. T
  d. F
  e. F

The RV is a smaller, thinner-walled and a more triangular-shaped cavity than the LV. The RV is anatomically situated anteriorly to the LV and is therefore closer to the chest wall. In the RV inflow view, it is the anterior and septal leaflets of the TV that are visualised. Various measurements of the RV have now been validated by the BSE, and RV dimensions should generally be measured in the apical 4-chamber view.

2 a. T
  b. T
  c. T
  d. T
  e. T

All are recognised causes of pulmonary arterial hypertension. Ischaemic heart disease causes LV systolic and diastolic dysfunction, which eventually causes raised LA pressures, leading to pulmonary hypertension. Both MR and MS cause the same. Connective tissue diseases such as SLE and systemic sclerosis affect the tunica layers of the pulmonary vascular bed causing increased resistance and raised pulmonary pressures. Chronic thromboembolic disease also causes resistance in the pulmonary vasculature, leading to increased PA pressures. Shunts such as VSDs and ASDs can also cause pulmonary hypertension.

3 a. F
  b. F
  c. T
  d. F
  e. T

TR may cause RV volume overload and dilatation, but does not generally produce pressure overload, which is more in keeping with RVH. ARVC causes hypokinesis and thinning of the RV free wall, often with localised aneurysms. PS causes pressure overload and RVH, akin to AS in the LV causing LVH. Aortic dissection does not cause RVH. In congenitally corrected transposition of the great vessels, the morphological RV becomes the systemic ventricle, leading to RVH.

4 a. T
  b. F
  c. F
  d. T
  e. T

Carcinoid heart disease is caused by metastatic carcinoid tumour to the liver, secreting 5-HT or serotonin products that affect right heart valves but are degraded in the lungs and do not therefore affect the left-sided valves (unless there is a right to left shunt). The TV is thickened and immobile in this condition. The commonest cardiac defect in Down's syndrome is a primum ASD or AVSD. The PV, not the TV, is harvested as part of the Ross procedure to replace the AV. Right-sided valves are more at risk of endocarditis in IV drug abusers. The TV is normally located slightly more apically than the MV.

5 a. T
  b. T
  c. T
  d. F
  e. F

Severe TR causes systolic flow reversal in the SVC and IVC. Physiological PR is well recognised and can be used to calculate the PA pressure in diastole. A TR jet velocity of 4.5 m/s indicates severe pulmonary hypertension and gives no indication of the severity or otherwise of the TR. Peak PA velocity is not used to calculate the systolic PA pressure because in pulmonary hypertension, there is no gradient between the RV and PA (assuming the PV is normal), only between the RV and RA.

6 a. T
  b. F
  c. T
  d. F
  e. T

PS is present in approximately 20% of patients with Noonan's syndrome. It is also well recognised with Tetralogy of Fallot (which also comprises RVH, overriding aorta and VSD) and Alagille's syndrome, a genetic, multisystem disorder affecting the liver and kidneys, as well as the heart. Transposition of the great vessels causes congenital cyanotic heart disease but PS is not a feature. Similarly, PS is not recognised with ARVC.

7 a. T
   b. T
   c. T
   d. T
   e. T

All are true according to BSE guidelines for RV measurement and assessment.

8 a. T
   b. T
   c. F
   d. T
   e. T

D-shaped septum in diastole only with normal septal movement in systole is caused by isolated RV volume overload, pushing the septum towards the LV in diastole, but the LV still controlling septal dynamics in systole. D-shaped septum in both systole and diastole suggests RV volume overload causing the diastolic shape and an element of pressure overload causing the RV to take over septal dynamics in systole. LBBB causes sudden, rapid downward septal motion on M-mode. A flat septum during systole and diastole implies LV and RV mass is equal such that neither ventricle controls septal motion any more than the other. Dilatation of the entire right heart with paradoxical septal motion should raise the possibility of a shunt at the atrial level, causing RV volume overload.

9 a. T
   b. T
   c. T
   d. T
   e. F

RV wall thickness of >0.5 cm suggests RVH. The normal end-diastolic diameter of the RV is 3.3 cm at mid-level in the apical 4-chamber view. The long-axis length can be up to 8 cm. Pulmonary hypertension causes the RV peak pressures to approximate LV pressures. The systolic PA Doppler waveform begins to look like that of the peak aortic waveform and there is an almost instantaneous rise to peak velocity (hence a short time to peak PA velocity of <80 ms). The IVRT of the RV is prolonged because the high PA pressures cause the PV to close earlier than normal. A PA diameter greater than the aorta suggests pulmonary hypertension, but a main PA diameter of >3 cm is also suggestive.

10 a. F
 b. T
 c. F
 d. F
 e. T

The likely diagnosis here is a PE. Using $4v^2$, the diastolic PA pressure (using the PR jet) is 36 mmHg and systolic pressure is 49 mmHg. But right atrial pressure must be added onto the latter. Using the IVC information, one should add an extra 10–15 mmHg to the 49 mmHg giving an estimated systolic PA pressure of 60–65 mmHg. With this degree of volume (and pressure) overload, the septal motion will be paradoxical and not normal. Thrombolysis of massive PE should be considered here.

11 a. T
 b. F
 c. F
 d. F
 e. T

RV systolic pressure and therefore PA systolic pressure (as there is no PS) can be calculated from the VSD jet in the absence of a TR jet. The inter-ventricular gradient is calculated by $4v^2$, which is 36 mmHg in this example. Knowing that the LV systolic pressure is 90 mmHg from the BP, the RV systolic pressure is 90 − 36 = 54 mmHg; although the IVC only minimally collapses on inspiration, indicating an estimated RA pressure of around 15–20 mmHg, this does not need to be added to the PA pressure as it is not being calculated from the TR jet, where RA pressure must be taken into account. Eisenmenger's syndrome occurs when pulmonary pressures are so high that there is shunt reversal, producing right to left flow; in this example, flow is clearly left to right. A D-shaped septum in diastole is in keeping with volume overload as is RV dilatation, but a flat septum in systole indicates a degree of pressure overload as well.

Volume overload of the RV is not caused by a VSD, as blood is shunted directly into the PA in systole and should prompt a search for another cause in the absence of TR, such as an ASD.

12 a. T
   b. F
   c. T
   d. T
   e. F

The moderator band is a prominent muscle trabeculation that carries the right bundle. It winds around the RV apex obliquely. The TV does have papillary muscles but the attachments are different to those of the MV and are delineated with far more difficulty on echo. The IVC enters the RA inferior to the coronary sinus and the crista terminalis traverses the anterior wall of the RA from the SVC towards it. The Eustachian valve is a residual embryonic attachment seen sometimes at the point of entry of the IVC into the RA. When this valve has a more extensive fenestration, it is termed the Chiari network. Both are considered normal variants.

13 a. T
   b. T
   c. F
   d. F
   e. T

The presence of a Chiari network is associated with an increased risk of ASD/PFO. Lushka's muscle is an accessory papillary muscle of the septal leaflet of the TV sometimes seen in the RVOT. The TR jet calculation may overestimate the PA pressure in PS and PA pressure in this instance should be calculated by $PAP = [[4(V_{TR})^2 + RAP]] - 4(V_{PS})^2$. Positive pressure ventilation changes the normally negative intra-thoracic pressures required to cause inspiration, therefore evaluation of the IVC collapse due to respiration is not helpful. The short time to peak velocity in the PA due to pulmonary hypertension is offset in RV dysfunction by the inability of the RV to contract sufficiently vigorously, causing the time to peak velocity to appear normal.

14 a. T
   b. T
   c. F

d. T

e. T

EF is normally 45 ± 5% for the RV. TAPSE is assessed using M-mode placed at the tricuspid annulus and measuring the forward displacement of annulus in systole. A displacement of <1.5 cm suggests RV dysfunction. RV function can also be measured using tissue Doppler techniques. The Tei index is (IVRT + IVCT) ÷ RV ejection duration.

15 a. T

b. T

c. T

d. F

e. T

ARVC causes fatty infiltration of the RV and sometimes the LV. Localised RV aneurysms are highly suggestive of the diagnosis. Tissue Doppler at the tricuspid annulus shows a positive velocity peak just before the onset of RV systole, which represents isovolumic contraction. As scarred segments of myocardium can be tethered and moved along with adjacent viable myocardium, measuring velocity with tissue Doppler is not as accurate an assessment of RV function as strain rate imaging, because the latter measures actual deformation of myocardium that therefore represents actively contracting myocardium only. A Tei index of <0.4 represents normal RV function. Albeit an unreliable sign, McConnell's sign, which is normal apical and mid-wall contraction of the RV with akinesis of the basal segment, is seen sometimes in large PEs. Unhelpfully, the reverse McConnell sign is also recognised in acute PEs.

16 a. T

b. F

c. F

d. T

e. F

Tamponade exaggerates the normal response to breathing, so that there is a decrease in transmitral flow in inspiration and an increase across the TV in inspiration. High right-sided pressures may mask features such as collapse of the RA and RV, as well as Doppler VTIs. ARVC is a rare cause of RWMA; ischaemic heart disease, PEs and bundle branch block are more common causes. A non-collapsing IVC during inspiration suggests an RA pressure of ≥20 mmHg. The Gerbode defect usually involves a shunt from the LV to the RA, not the RV to the LA.

17 a. T
   b. F
   c. T
   d. F
   e. F

As PA pressure rises, the Doppler profile begins to resemble aortic flow with a mid-systolic notch similar to the dicrotic notch seen in normal aortic flow. As PA diastolic pressure also rises, the PV will close increasingly earlier. A PR jet velocity of 1.5 m/s indicates a diastolic PA pressure of around 9 mmHg. Severe TR does not necessarily suggest pulmonary hypertension, as it may be functional or secondary to primary valve pathology. A peak systolic PA velocity of 4 m/s suggests PS; PA pressure may be normal.

18 a. F
   b. F
   c. T
   d. F
   e. F

In the 4-chamber view, base to apex of up to 7.9 cm is considered normal whereas >9 cm would be considered severe dilatation. A basal diameter of >4 cm suggests severe dilatation. A PISA radius of >0.9 cm indicates severe TR and a regurgitant fraction of >60% indicates severe PR. Dilated hepatic veins usually occur when RA pressure has reached at least 15 mmHg.

19 a. F
   b. F
   c. T
   d. T
   e. F

LV involvement due to ARVC is recognised but uncommon. Restrictive cardiomyopathies, particularly infiltrative aetiologies such as amyloid, affect both the RV and LV. Like LBBB, RBBB also produces septal dyssynchrony. The normal position of the TV is more apical than the MV. RV pacing leads are increasingly placed in the RVOT septum to produce more physiological pacing.

20 a. T
   b. F
   c. F

d. T

e. T

Using tissue Doppler, a systolic velocity of the tricuspid annulus of >10 cm/s is considered normal. The Simpson's method is limited to single plane when assessing RV EF, which is normally about 45%. Myxomas are rare but do occur in the right heart. Right atrial area by planimetry should measure <20 cm^2 if normal and tricuspid stenosis is indeed rare, occurring almost solely due to rheumatic disease.

6 Prosthetic Valves and Endocarditis

QUESTIONS

For each question below, decide whether the answers provided are true or false.

1 The following are true of prosthetic valves:
   a. The St. Jude's mechanical valve is a single leaflet valve
   b. The Starr–Edwards valve is rarely used now for valve replacements
   c. Stentless bioprostheses have a more physiological haemodynamic profile
   d. Replacement valve effective orifice areas are smaller than a normal native valve
   e. Aortic prostheses can now be implanted percutaneously

2 The following can be normal echocardiographic features when assessing prosthetic valves:
   a. Two forward jets in colour Doppler when a bileaflet prosthesis opens
   b. No regurgitant jets when a bileaflet prosthesis closes
   c. Forward flow through a mitral prosthesis directed antero-medially
   d. Antegrade velocities of 2–3 m/s through aortic prostheses
   e. Significant reverberation artefact with mechanical valves

3 The following statements are true:
   a. TOE removes the problem of acoustic shadowing when assessing a prosthetic AV
   b. Porcine valves are used as AVRs in the Ross procedure
   c. Paraprosthetic regurgitation suggests dehiscence

Successful Accreditation in Echocardiography: A Self-Assessment Guide,
First Edition. Sanjay M. Banypersad and Keith Pearce.
© 2012 John Wiley & Sons, Ltd. Published 2012 by John Wiley & Sons, Ltd.

d. Pannus can lead to valve dysfunction

e. Bioprosthetic valve failure is common after 3 years of implantation

4 The following are true:

   a. There are more mechanical than bioprosthetic valve replacements per year in the UK

   b. Mechanical valves require serial echocardiographic follow-up

   c. Velocity ratio can be useful in serial assessment of prosthetic AV function

   d. Persistent LVH post AVR can sometimes be due to patient–prosthesis mismatch

   e. Tissue valve replacements can become calcified with time

5 When performing echo to assess prosthetic MV dysfunction:

   a. TTE has a high negative predictive value

   b. The pressure half-time method is not useful for serial follow-up of mitral prostheses

   c. Antegrade velocities are higher than native valves

   d. Spontaneous echo contrast in the LV always suggests a low-flow state

   e. The apical 4-chamber view is generally the most helpful for assessing prosthetic MVs

6 The following are true when assessing prosthetic valve dysfunction:

   a. Recurrence of pulmonary hypertension suggests prosthetic MV dysfunction

   b. Infected pannus is similar in appearance to thrombus

   c. Root abscesses may be echo-lucent or echo-dense

   d. Peak gradient across a prosthetic AVR of 30 mmHg is always abnormal

   e. The finding of vegetations always represents acute infection

7 When assessing prosthetic valve dysfunction:

   a. Peak E inflow velocity is not useful when assessing prosthetic MV stenosis

   b. Washing jets, if seen, are abnormal

   c. A 29 mm Medtronic–Hall aortic prosthesis would be expected to have a peak velocity of 3.3 m/s

   d. Paravalvular leaks are not subject to the Choanda effect

   e. Tissue valves may be manufactured from animal pericardium

8 The following are strongly suggestive of severe prosthetic aortic valve dysfunction:
  a. Regurgitant volume of 45 ml
  b. Regurgitant jet width/LVOT area ratio of 70%
  c. Diastolic flow reversal in the abdominal aorta
  d. Two symmetrical transvalvular regurgitant jets through a Starr–Edwards prosthesis
  e. LVOT:Aortic VTI ratio >0.3

9 The following are strongly suggestive of mitral prosthetic dysfunction:
  a. Regurgitant orifice area of 0.5 cm^2
  b. Regurgitant fraction of 60%
  c. Peak E velocity of 2 m/s
  d. Vena contracta <0.3 cm
  e. LA of 5.7 cm

10 In a patient with endocarditis, the following might be found on echocardiography:
  a. Vegetations
  b. Paravalvular abscess
  c. LV thrombus
  d. Janeway lesions
  e. Pericardial effusion

11 The following echocardiographic findings are major criteria for the diagnosis of endocarditis:
  a. New valvular regurgitation
  b. Oscillating mass on an annuloplasty ring
  c. Pericardial effusion
  d. New prosthetic valve dehiscence
  e. LV aneurysm

12 Endocarditis should be considered when performing echocardiography in febrile patients with a history of the following:
  a. Cardiac transplantation
  b. IV drug abusers
  c. Congenital heart disease
  d. Prosthetic valves
  e. Pacing lead in situ

13 The following are true of endocarditis:
- **a.** Organisms found on the skin are the commonest cause of prosthetic valve endocarditis within the first year
- **b.** Any part of a valve leaflet may be affected
- **c.** In most cases, endocarditis affects a previously abnormal valve
- **d.** Large, highly mobile vegetations should be considered for urgent surgery
- **e.** Libman–Sachs endocarditis is caused by fungi

14 The following are true of vegetations:
- **a.** Rapidly oscillate
- **b.** Are also commonly seen in acute rheumatic fever
- **c.** Their motion is dependent on valve motion but more chaotic
- **d.** Can appear similar to Lambl's excrescences in suspected AV endocarditis
- **e.** In MV endocarditis would be expected to be attached to the left ventricular side of the valve

15 The following are true of endocarditis:
- **a.** The negative predictive value of TOE is better than TTE in endocarditis
- **b.** AV vegetations are more readily identified on parasternal views than apical views
- **c.** M-Mode is not useful in assessing endocarditis
- **d.** MV endocarditis can spread to involve the AV
- **e.** There is a predominance of left-sided endocarditis in IV drug abusers

16 The following can mimic the appearance of a vegetation:
- **a.** Beam-width artefact
- **b.** Flail MV leaflet
- **c.** Quadricuspid AV
- **d.** Excessive suture material
- **e.** Ruptured papillary muscle

17 Complications of endocarditis include:
- **a.** Leaflet perforation
- **b.** Valvular regurgitation
- **c.** Valvular stenosis
- **d.** Aneurysm of the sinus of valsalva
- **e.** Thrombotic vegetations

18 The following is true of infective endocarditis affecting the TV:
   a. Has a worse prognosis than left-sided valve disease
   b. Can lead to septic pulmonary emboli
   c. TOE is almost always required to be diagnostic
   d. Smoking cannabis increases the risk of developing it
   e. Can be caused by the carcinoid syndrome

19 The following are true regarding endocarditis:
   a. Blood culture results qualify as both major and minor Duke's criteria
   b. A papillary fibroelastoma may be confused with a vegetation
   c. Fungal endocarditis is typically associated with very small vegetations
   d. Pseudoaneurysm of the MV leaflet is a recognised complication of MV endocarditis
   e. All of the above

20 The following are true of an aortic root abscess:
   a. Is associated with 1st degree heart block
   b. Can rupture from the abscess cavity into the LV
   c. Can rupture from the LVOT into the RV
   d. Can rupture from the LVOT into the RA
   e. Systolic and diastolic Doppler flow from left to right suggests rupture at a level above the AV into the right heart

Prosthetic Valves and Endocarditis

ANSWERS

1 a. F
  b. T
  c. T
  d. T
  e. T

The St. Jude's valve is a bileaflet mechanism whereas Bjork Shiley is a single, tilting leaflet prosthesis. The Starr–Edwards valve is a 'ball and cage' mechanism and is very rarely used in valve surgery today. Bioprosthetic valves can be stented or stentless, the latter being haemodynamically more physiological but technically more complex to implant. Effective orifice areas are usually smaller than a normal native valve because of the support structures. Percutaneous AV implants are being increasingly performed in patients where open surgical replacement is deemed too high risk.

2 a. F
  b. F
  c. T
  d. T
  e. T

There are generally three antegrade jets seen on colour Doppler with a bileaflet prosthesis – one thin, central, high-velocity jet with two surrounding lateral jets as the two leaflets open. When they close, regurgitant jets are seen at the closure lines. Forward flow through the native MV is towards the apex, however, with most prosthetic valves, flow is directed antero-medially towards the ventricular septum. Depending on the size of the aortic prosthesis, CW velocities of up to 3 m/s can be normal with smaller prostheses. Transthoracic imaging of mechanical valves is often limited by acoustic shadowing and reverberation.

3 a. F
  b. F

c. T
d. T
e. F

TOE scanning of the AVR places the posterior aspect of the sewing ring in the near field of the remainder of the prosthesis, which may be obscured from view; this is not the case in the mitral position, where the acoustic shadowing affects the LV and therefore regurgitation into the LA can be appreciated. The Ross procedure harvests the native PV as the AVR. Paraprosthetic regurgitation is often seen in endocarditis causing valve dehiscence. Pannus formation is a well recognised cause of valve dysfunction, often by obstructing valve opening or closure. Bioprosthetic valves generally last up to 10 years post implantation before dysfunction becomes apparent.

4 a. T
  b. F
  c. T
  d. T
  e. T

Approximately 60–70% of artificial heart valve implants in the UK are mechanical, the remainder being either bioprosthetic or tissue. Mechanical valves should be routinely assessed after implantation but in the absence of symptoms or signs of suspected valve dysfunction do not require echocardiographic follow-up. Velocity ratios are useful in serial assessing aortic prostheses as they are not dependent on volume flow rate and do not require measurement of the LVOT. Patient–prosthesis mismatch in the aortic position can have a number of consequences, including raised resting and exertional gradients leading to persistence of LVH post surgery. Tissue valve replacements are subject to the same calcification processes as native valves.

5 a. F
  b. F
  c. T
  d. F
  e. F

The absence of MR on a transthoracic study does not rule out prosthetic MV dysfunction because of problems with acoustic shadowing and reverberations, therefore TTE has a low negative predictive value. Although the rate of decline of the peak velocity (i.e. pressure half time) is not affected by prosthetic valves, the Hatle equation is only derived for native valves. Thus, valve area calculations are not valid, but serial pressure half-time measurements can still be useful. Antegrade velocities are higher than in native valves because of the presence of the sewing ring. Spontaneous echo contrast can be seen in the LV because of microcavitation due to the occluder opening and closing and does not necessarily always represent a low-flow state. The apical 4-chamber view is often the least helpful for assessing MVs as reverberation from the prosthesis obscures the LA.

6 a. T
  b. T
  c. T
  d. F
  e. F

Pulmonary hypertension, which resolves following MV surgery and then recurs, is suggestive of dysfunction of the MV prosthesis. Infected pannus from endocarditis has a similar echodensity to thrombus. Abscesses may be echolucent or echo dense. A peak gradient of 30 mmHg across a prosthetic AVR may be normal for a small-sized prosthesis. Vegetations can represent prior endocarditis that is not actively infective (i.e. healed), as well as acute infection; the clinical picture should dictate.

7 a. F
  b. F
  c. F
  d. F
  e. T

Peak E velocity of >2–2.5 m/s depending on valve type can be suggestive of narrowing of the MV orifice. Washing jets are normal and prevent clot from forming on the prostheses. A 29 mm single-tilting disc in the aortic position would be expected to have a peak velocity of around 1.9 m/s. Paravalvular leaks are subject to the Choanda effect as the jets are close to chamber walls, producing eccentric jets. Ionescu–Shiley prostheses are derived from bovine pericardium.

8 a. F
  b. T
  c. T
  d. F
  e. F

A regurgitant volume of >60 ml and a jet width/LVOT ratio of >65% are in keeping with severe prosthetic regurgitation. Diastolic flow reversal in the abdominal aorta suggests significant regurgitation. Two small symmetrical transvalvular regurgitant jets through a Starr–Edwards prosthesis may be normal. A VTI ratio of >0.3 suggests no significant stenosis.

9 a. T
  b. T
  c. F
  d. F
  e. F

A regugitant orifice area of >0.4 cm^2 and a regurgitant fraction of >50% both represent severe MR and therefore severe prosthetic MV dysfunction. A peak E velocity of 2 m/s is not necessarily strongly suggestive of mitral prosthetic dysfunction; it may be normal for the St. Jude's or Starr–Edwards prostheses or may represent increased cardiac output from fever or IV fluids. A vena contracta of <0.3 cm indicates minimal MR. A LA of 5.7 cm is significantly dilated but does not strongly suggests valve dysfunction as dilated LA can persist from pre-surgery or simply represent chronic AF.

10 a. T
  b. T
  c. F
  d. F
  e. T

Vegetations and abscesses are classic features of endocarditis. Thrombus occurs in areas of akinesia, commonly seen in ischaemic or dilated cardiomyopathies rather than endocarditis. Janeway lesions are found on the hands in endocarditis and are not therefore detectable on echocardiography. A pericardial effusion can be seen in endocarditis and can be reactive or septic.

11 a. T
  b. T
  c. F
  d. T
  e. F

In addition to the above, Modified Duke's major criteria also include two positive blood cultures for a typical organism, or two positive blood cultures ≥12 h apart of an organism consistent with endocarditis, or one positive blood culture for *Coxiella Burnettii*. Pericardial effusions and LV aneurysms do not form any part of the Modified Duke's Critera; LV aneurysms are not a feature of endocarditis.

12 a. T
  b. T
  c. T
  d. T
  e. T
All are predisposing factors for endocarditis.

13 a. T
  b. T
  c. T
  d. T
  e. F
The commonest cause of native valve endocarditis is *Streptococcus viridans*. The commonest cause of prosthetic valve endocarditis within the first 6–12 months of implant is coagulase-negative Staphylococci, such as *Staphylococcus epidermidis*. Any part of the native valve leaflet may be affected but it is commonly the coaptation line. Endocarditis usually affects a valve that is abnormal in the first place. Large (>1–1.5 cm), highly mobile vegetations are most at risk of embolism and should therefore be referred urgently for surgical assessment. Libman–Sachs endocarditis is caused by SLE and not by fungi.

14 a. T
  b. F
  c. T
  d. T
  e. F
Vegetations are irregular, echogenic masses whose movement is chaotic and dependent on valve motion (i.e. aortic vegetations prolapse into the LVOT in diastole and into aorta in systole), but often excessively and chaotically with rapid oscillations in diastole. Vegetations are not commonly seen in acute rheumatic fever as the pathophysiology is immune-complex cross-reactivity causing inflammation of valve tissue, rather than a true infective process as in endocarditis. Lambl's excrescences are filaments attached to the AV and are sometimes confused with other pathologies such as endocarditis. In MV endocarditis, the vegetation would be expected

to be attached to the left atrial side of the MV and in AV endocarditis, would be attached to the left ventricular side of the valve.

15 a. T
  b. T
  c. F
  d. T
  e. F

A negative TTE does not exclude a diagnosis of endocarditis if it is clinically strongly suspected and TOE is usually indicated in that scenario. Parasternal views are generally better at identifying AV vegetations. M-Mode can be very useful in assessing rapid oscillatory motion of masses in suspected endocarditis. Fibrous continuity between the MV and AV means infection can spread easily to involve both valves. IV drug abusers tend to have more right-sided endocarditis.

16 a. T
  b. T
  c. T
  d. T
  e. T

All can give the appearance of a mobile mass attached to a valve.

17 a. T
  b. T
  c. T
  d. T
  e. T

Vegetations can disrupt the coaptation line or simply destroy the leaflet leading to perforation. Rarely, stenosis can result from a large vegetation obstructing the opening of the orifice. A sinus of valsalva aneurysm can occur as a result of extension of infection from the AV causing wall thinning and dilatation at the level of the sinus of valsalva. Vegetations composed of fibrin and platelets, rather than bacteria, can occur in marantic endocarditis.

18 a. F
  b. T
  c. F
  d. F
  e. F

Right-sided endocarditis generally has a more favourable prognosis than left-sided endocarditis. Systemic embolic activity is not seen as vegetations lodge in the pulmonary vasculature and may cause septic pulmonary emboli, however bacteria can still enter the systemic circulation through the pulmonary bed. The TV is close to the chest wall and therefore TTE is usually diagnostic. Injection of IV substances increases the risk of staphylococcal bacteria entering the venous blood; smoking cannabis does not. Tricuspid endocarditis is not caused by the carcinoid syndrome but carcinoid is a rare but well recognised cause of right-sided valvular thickening and regurgitation; PS is also seen.

19 a. T
   b. T
   c. F
   d. T
   e. F

Positive blood cultures can be a major or a minor criterion depending on the type of organism cultured and time between each culture. Numerous abnormalities may be mistaken for vegetations including papillary fibroelastoma, nodules of Arantius and myxomatous leaflets. Fungal endocarditis and the *Haemophilus influenza* bacterium are associated with large vegetations. A pseudo-aneurysm of the MV leaflet is an uncommon but recognised complication of mitral endocarditis.

20 a. T
   b. T
   c. T
   d. T
   e. T

Aortic root abscesses are in close proximity to the conduction tissue and can cause 1st degree heart block. Rupture is possible in a number of ways. The abscess cavity can rupture into the LV showing colour Doppler flow into and out of the cavity. It can also rupture from the LVOT into either the RV (causing a VSD) or across the atrioventricular septum into the RA causing a Gerbode defect. Rupture in the aortic outflow tract at the level of the sinus of valsalva into the RV would show Doppler flow from left to right in both systole and diastole.

7 Pericardial Disease and Cardiac Masses

QUESTIONS

For each question below, decide whether the answers provided are true or false.

1 The following are true of atrial myxomas:
  a. More frequently arise from the RA than the LA
  b. Are the commonest benign cardiac tumour
  c. Readily embolise
  d. Commonly invade adjacent tissues
  e. Can range from 1–15 cm in diameter

2 With regard to atrial myxomas:
  a. They can be seen to prolapse through the MV
  b. They can occur on the MV
  c. Classically attach via a stalk to the atrial septum
  d. Can recur after resection
  e. Can be familial when part of the Carney syndrome

3 The following are true of thrombus:
  a. May be seen in the atrial appendage in AF
  b. Can occur in regions of akinesia in the LV
  c. Should be suspected when spontaneous echo contrast is seen in the LV
  d. Can be seen with apical aneurysms
  e. Can be seen with pseudo-aneurysms of the LV

4 The following increase the risk of thrombus formation:
  a. MR
  b. Pacing wire

Successful Accreditation in Echocardiography: A Self-Assessment Guide,
First Edition. Sanjay M. Banypersad and Keith Pearce.
© 2012 John Wiley & Sons, Ltd. Published 2012 by John Wiley & Sons, Ltd.

    c. Central lines
    d. Rheumatic MS
    e. AS

5 The following statements are true regarding cardiac masses:
    a. Renal cancers may extend as one complete mass from the kidney to the RA
    b. Sarcomas are the most common primary malignant tumour
    c. Carcinoid tumours commonly metastasise to right-sided valves
    d. Uterine tumours extend up the IVC to the RA similar to renal tumours
    e. Metastases to the pericardium are a recognised complication of melanomas

6 The following is true of papillary fibroelastomas:
    a. Most commonly arise from the posterior wall of the atrium
    b. Have a similar appearance to lipomatous hypertrophy of the atrial septum
    c. Are similar to vegetations in that they occur on the upstream side of the valve
    d. Are frequently embolic
    e. Invasion of the pericardium with a pericardial effusion would be expected

7 The following are true of sarcomas:
    a. Preferentially affect the RA
    b. Have smooth borders similar to myxomas
    c. May arise from the inter-atrial septum
    d. Are associated with a pericardial effusion
    e. CT/MRI is often required for tissue characterisation

8 The following predispose to left ventricular thrombus:
    a. Dilated cardiomyopathy
    b. Apical infarct
    c. Hypereosinophilic syndrome
    d. Pseudo-aneurysm
    e. All of the above

9 In pericardial constriction, the following features are usually seen:
    a. Biatrial enlargement
    b. Normal EF

    c. Left ventricular hypertrophy

    d. Increased reversal of SVC flow during expiration

    e. Shortened MV deceleration time

10 Pericardial effusions are best visualised/diagnosed in the following views:

    a. Suprasternal

    b. Parasternal short axis

    c. Parasternal long axis

    d. Subcostal window

    e. Apical 2-chamber view

11 The following features are consistent when diagnosing cardiac tamponade due to a large pericardial effusion:

    a. Breathlessness usually with congested lungs

    b. Bradycardia

    c. Hypertension

    d. Elevated jugular venous pressure

    e. Loud heart sounds

12 When considering respiratory variation in cardiac tamponade, the following statements are true:

    a. Tricuspid E wave variation >25%

    b. Mitral E wave variation <15%

    c. Peak LVOT velocity and VTI variation >10%

    d. Peak RVOT velocity and VTI variation <10%

    e. Peak aortic CW Doppler velocity variation >25%

13 With reference to tumours of the heart:

    a. Metastatic tumours of the heart are more common than primary tumours

    b. Metastatic tumours typically involve the pericardium

    c. Metastatic tumours typically involve the endocardium

    d. The most common echo finding suggesting metastasis is valvular thickening

    e. Those tumours with the greatest propensity to metastasise to the heart are melanomas

14 Features consistent with pericardial effusion:

    a. Ends anterior to descending aorta

    b. Almost never overlaps the RA

    c. Rarely >4 cm in depth

  d. Heart is fixed in one position
  e. All of the above

15 The following statements are true regarding pericardial disease:
  a. Calcification of the pericardium can be seen in patients with previous TB infection
  b. Constriction can be a consequence of previous pericarditis
  c. Constriction leads to diastolic equalisation of pressures in all cardiac chambers
  d. Pericardial effusions are commonly seen with amyloidosis
  e. In constriction, the ventricular septum shows signs of ventricular interdependence during respiration

16 In congenital absence of the pericardium, the following statements are true:
  a. The RV will appear enlarged in the parasternal window
  b. Is associated with bronchogenic cysts
  c. Is associated with an ASD
  d. Is associated with a bicuspid aortic valve
  e. Usually involves absence of the right-sided pericardium

17 With reference to pericardiocentesis via the subcostal route:
  a. Must always be performed using echo guidance
  b. Agitated saline must never be used
  c. Usually promotes tachycardia during aspiration
  d. Reduction in fluid cavity on echo is immediately seen
  e. Loculated effusions will add to the risk of pericardial puncture

18 The following features favour the diagnosis of pericardial constriction over restriction:
  a. Diastolic dysfunction
  b. A septal 'bounce' with respiration
  c. Calcified pericardium
  d. Respiratory variation in ventricular filling patterns on Doppler
  e. RA dilatation

19 When assessing a cardiac mass by echo:
  a. The presence of an RA mass should prompt IVC interrogation
  b. The size of the mass determines aetiology

    c. Trans-pulmonary contrast can help differentiate tumour from thrombus

    d. Extracardiac compression never occurs without the presence of a pericardial collection

    e. The use of agitated saline is recommended

20 With reference to primary cardiac tumours in adults:

    a. Lipoma is the most common benign tumour

    b. Mesothelioma of the AV node is a benign tumour

    c. Rhabdomyosarcoma is the commonest malignant tumour

    d. Papillary fibroelastomas account for 10% of benign tumours

    e. Angiosarcomas are more common than fibrosarcomas

Pericardial Disease and Cardiac Masses

ANSWERS

1 a. F
   b. T
   c. T
   d. F
   e. T

Atrial myxomas usually arise in the LA, although occurrence in the RA is also recognised. They are the commonest type of benign cardiac tumour however, cardiac metastases from elsewhere are overall the most common type of tumour seen in the heart. Myxomas readily embolise, a common form of presentation, but rarely invade into local tissues. Significant variation in size is seen.

2 a. T
   b. T
   c. T
   d. T
   e. T

Myxomas attach via a stalk to the fossa ovalis of the atrial septum and can sometimes be seen to prolapse through the MV orifice. They can recur after resection due to the multicenteric nature of the disease rather than inadequate resection. Approximately 5–10% of myxomas occur as part of the Carney syndrome, which is also associated with thyroid and pituitary tumours. Occurrence on valves is very rare but described.

3 a. T
   b. T
   c. T
   d. T
   e. T

AF predisposes to thrombus formation in the atrium and atrial appendage. Thrombus can occur in the LV in regions of akinesia or significant hypokinesia such as in the apex following an apical infarct. Aneurysms are also likely to contain thrombus and pseudo-aneurysms are also often lined with thrombus. Spontaneous echo contrast should alert sonographers to the presence of a low-flow state predisposing to thrombus formation.

4 a. F
 b. T
 c. T
 d. T
 e. F

It is thought that mitral regurgitation encourages the 'washing-away' of thrombus from the LA and therefore the risk is not increased. However, rheumatic MS carries a high risk of thrombus formation even when in sinus rhythm. Pacing wires and central lines are all potential sources of thrombus formation in the right heart. AS does not carry an increased risk of cardiac thrombus formation.

5 a. T
 b. T
 c. F
 d. T
 e. T

Both renal and uterine cancers can extend up the IVC en masse to the RA. This is important to note as curative resection is possible in this situation. Malignant metastases are the commonest tumours found in the heart but sarcomas are the commonest *primary* malignant cardiac tumour. Myxomas are the most common benign cardiac tumours. Carcinoid tumours do not readily metastasise to right-sided heart valves – they secrete biologically active metabolites that fibrose and stiffen the valves. Melanomas have the highest rate of pericardial metastases.

6 a. F
 b. F
 c. F
 d. F
 e. F

Papillary fibroelastomas occur on valves, most commonly the MV. In this respect, they are not similar to lipomatous hypertrophy of the inter-atrial septum and do not commonly occur on the posterior wall. Although their motion may be similar to vegetations, their point of attachment is generally on the downstream side of the valve not the upstream side. They are benign tumours that do not generally embolise, unlike myxomas.

7 a. T
   b. F
   c. T
   d. T
   e. T

Sarcomas have a predilection for the RA but do occur in the LA. They are sometimes described as a 'cauliflower' mass due to their irregular borders. They can arise from the inter-atrial septum and extend into the atrial appendage. They can invade myocardium and pericardium, leading to a pericardial effusion. Most cardiac masses go on to be further characterised with CT or usually MRI.

8 a. T
   b. T
   c. F
   d. T
   e. F

Dilated cardiomyopathies generally lead to thinned myocardium and global hypokinesia, which is a substrate for thrombus formation. An apical infarct also causes apical wall motion abnormalities where there will be stasis of blood and thrombus formation. The hypereosinophilic syndrome is a multisystem disorder causing neurological as well as cardiac sequelae. Restrictive features and LV thrombus are well recognised. An LV pseudo-aneurysm is often lined with thrombus.

9 a. F
   b. T
   c. F
   d. T
   e. T

Biatrial enlargement is usually seen in RCM and not in pericardial constriction. The EF is usually normal, and LVH is more commonly seen in restriction. The SVC flow reversal is more dominant during expiration and shortening of the MV deceleration time is seen in both restriction and constriction.

10 a. F
  b. T
  c. T
  d. T
  e. F

Parasternal short-axis view is actually very useful sometimes for looking at posterior effusions and also for guiding drainage from the anterior intercostal approach. Parasternal long-axis, subcostal and apical 4-chamber views are also useful. Suprasternal and apical 2-chamber views are generally not useful for assessing pericardial effusions.

11 a. F
  b. F
  c. F
  d. T
  e. F

Patients are often breathless although have clear lungs. The patients usually have a tachycardia associated with hypotension. The JVP is elevated due to diastolic compression of the right heart and the heart sounds are quiet as a result of the pericardial effusion.

12 a. T
  b. F
  c. T
  d. F
  e. F

Tricuspid E-wave size will vary by greater than 25%. The MV E-wave size will vary by >15% and both LVOT and RVOT peak velocities and VTIs will vary by >10%. The aortic CW Doppler offers no clinical guide in the diagnosis of cardiac tamponade.

13 a. T
  b. T
  c. F
  d. F
  e. T

Metastatic tumours are more commonly found in the heart when compared with primary tumours, and they usually involve the pericardium and rarely involve the endocardium. The most commonly associated echo feature is a pericardial effusion and up to 65% of melanomas can metastasise to the heart.

14 a. T
   b. F
   c. T
   d. F
   e. F

The pericardial fluid ends anteriorly to the descending aorta and is best visualised in the parasternal long-axis view. Pericardial fluid will overlap the RA and does not usually overlap the LA. A pericardial effusion does not usually exceed 4 cm in depth. The heart is usually hypermobile within a pericardial collection.

15 a. T
   b. T
   c. T
   d. T
   e. T

TB is a recognised cause of calcification in various parts of the body, including the pericardium. Pericarditis, uraemia and connective tissue disorders are some of the causes of pericardial constriction that classically leads to equalisation of diastolic pressures in all cardiac chambers; this can be demonstrated at cardiac catheterisation. Pericardial effusions are common in cardiac amyloidosis, along with valve thickening and LV thickening, with small ventricles and large atria. A septal 'bounce' due to ventricular interdependence is a characteristic finding in constrictive pericarditis.

16 a. T
   b. T
   c. T
   d. T
   e. F

The entire cardiac structure is shifted towards the left, resulting in the appearance of RV volume overload in the standard parasternal views. Bronchogenic cysts, ASD and bicuspid AVs are all associated with this condition. Absence of the left-sided pericardium is more common.

17 a. F
   b. F
   c. F
   d. T
   e. T

Pericardiocentesis can be performed using echo or fluoroscopy; indeed, it is sometimes performed blind in emergency situations. Agitated saline can be used to confirm the needle is in the pericardial space (and not the RV) before advancing the guidewire. Slowing of the tachycardia usually results when pericardial fluid is removed, and the echo appearances are seen immediately. Loculated effusions may increase the possibility of pericardial puncture.

18 a. F
   b. T
   c. T
   d. T
   e. F

Diastolic dysfunction is common to both, although in RCM is due to myocardial stiffening and in constriction is due to non-compliant pericardium. A septal 'bounce' with respiration occurs due to ventricular interdependence in constriction, and is not a feature of restriction. A calcified pericardium suggests constriction and respiratory variation on Doppler filling patterns across the atrioventricular valves is also consistent. RA dilatation is not considered definitive in the differentiation of the restriction/constriction.

19 a. T
   b. F
   c. T
   d. F
   e. F

RA masses can result from direct metastasis from hepatomas and hypernephromas via the IVC. The mass size does not determine aetiology but may assist the chosen method of extraction. Transpulmonary contrast may help if there is a rich blood supply to the cardiac tumour; agitated saline will not assist in differentiation. Extracardiac masses can be visible without evidence of pericardial collection, e.g. coronary aneurysm, hiatus hernia.

20 a. F
   b. T
   c. F
   d. T
   e. T

The most common benign primary cardiac tumour is a myxoma (27%). Lipomas and papillary fibroelastomas account for 10% each, mesothelioma of the AV node accounts for 1% of benign tumours; angiosarcomas are the commonest primary malignant tumour (9%) with rhabdomyosarcomas accounting for 5% and fibrosarcomas for 3%.

8 Adult Congenital Heart Disease

QUESTIONS

For each question below, decide whether the answers provided are true or false.

1 The following are true of Ebstein's anomaly:
   a. Causes a dilated RA
   b. Commonly leads to malignant tumours in later life
   c. The TV is more basally displaced than the MV
   d. Is associated with an ASD
   e. Is associated with severe tricuspid stenosis

2 During echocardiography of a patient with a Fontan's circulation:
   a. A single functioning ventricle is expected
   b. The PA may be connected directly to the RA
   c. The PA may be connected directly to the IVC
   d. Arrhythmias are generally well tolerated
   e. Dehydration is generally poorly tolerated

3 In a patient with surgically corrected transposition of the great vessels, the following may be found on echo:
   a. An ASD may be found
   b. Intra-atrial baffles may be seen
   c. The RV is always the systemic ventricle
   d. The pulmonary veins are detached from the LA and attached to the RA
   e. The patient may be cyanosed

Successful Accreditation in Echocardiography: A Self-Assessment Guide,
First Edition. Sanjay M. Banypersad and Keith Pearce.
© 2012 John Wiley & Sons, Ltd. Published 2012 by John Wiley & Sons, Ltd.

4 In a patient with congenitally corrected transposition of the great vessels:
   a. The moderator band is in the LV
   b. The PA exits the LV
   c. The SVC drains into the LA
   d. VSD is essential in order to be compatible with life
   e. The MV is attached to the RV

5 With regard to ASDs:
   a. Ostium secundum is the commonest type
   b. The apical 4-chamber view is the optimal view for detecting defects
   c. They cause right-sided dilatation
   d. Sinus venosus defects are associated with anomalous pulmonary venous drainage
   e. Ostium secundum cases can be closed percutaneously in many cases

6 When performing echocardiography in an asymptomatic adult with a PDA:
   a. There is usually a significant right-to-left shunt
   b. LA and LV dilatation may be seen
   c. RA and RV dilatation is seen as the shunt is left to right
   d. Diastolic flow reversal in the descending aorta similar to AR may be seen
   e. In utero, the PDA causes blood to bypass the lungs

7 The following are true of VSDs:
   a. Perimembranous defects are the commonest
   b. Inlet VSDs may be associated with AVSDs
   c. Cause right ventricular dilatation if the shunt is left to right
   d. A high velocity CW Doppler signal would be expected with a small VSD
   e. A ventricular septal aneurysm is suggestive of previous spontaneously closed VSD

8 The following are true of coarctations of the aorta:
   a. Is a recognised cause of hypertension
   b. If severe, causes diastolic flow reversal on Doppler
   c. Leads to BP differences between the upper and lower body
   d. Imaging with CT is generally superior to echo
   e. Can be associated with bicuspid AVs

9 The following are true of PFOs:
  a. Cause right-sided dilatation
  b. Allow continuous right-to-left flow in utero
  c. Allow continuous left-to-right flow in adulthood
  d. Are a potential cause of cryptogenic stroke in adulthood
  e. Valsalva with injection of agitated saline through an antecubital vein is the best method for demonstrating the presence of a PFO

10 The following features might be seen in uncorrected Tetralogy of Fallot:
  a. A high peak RVOT velocity
  b. Dilated PA
  c. VSD with left-to-right flow
  d. Thinning of the RV free wall
  e. VSD with right-to-left flow

11 The following are true of Tetralogy of Fallot:
  a. The VSD is generally of the muscular type
  b. Anomalous coronary artery anatomy can be associated
  c. Pulmonary stenosis can be protective against developing pulmonary hypertension
  d. Can be surgically palliated by the Blalock–Taussig shunt
  e. The origin of the aortic root is anteriorly displaced causing an overriding aorta

12 The following are true of intra-cardiac shunts when performing echocardiography in ACHD patients:
  a. A Glenn shunt connects the SVC to the PA
  b. A Potts shunt connects the descending aorta to the left PA
  c. The Blalock–Taussig shunt connects the subclavian vein to the PA
  d. The Waterston shunt connects the ascending aorta to the right PA
  e. Shunts are sometimes removed at the time of corrective surgery

13 In ACHD echocardiography, the following procedures may have been performed in childhood for the following conditions:
  a. The Rastelli procedure for transposition of the great vessels and a VSD

b. The Fontan procedure for single ventricle systems

c. The Norwood procedure for single ventricle systems

d. Damus–Kaye–Stansel procedure for Ebstein's anomaly

e. The Konno procedure for congenital PS

14 You perform an echocardiogram on a 30-year-old male with breathlessness. In addition to a volume overloaded right heart, you also find LVOT diameter 2.1 cm, VTI_{LVOT} 18 cm, RVOT diameter 2.8 cm, VTI_{RVOT} 36 cm, peak RVOT velocity 1.9 m/s, peak PA velocity 3.3 m/s. IVC collapses normally. The following are true:

a. The PA systolic pressure can be calculated from the data above

b. An ASD is the likely cause

c. A VSD is the likely cause

d. The $Q_p : Q_s$ shunt calculation is approximately 3.5:1

e. A degree of PS is present

15 In the presence of a bicuspid AV, the following statements are true:

a. Familial screening is recommended

b. Some degree of prolapse is seen in 5–10% of patients

c. VSDs are a well-recognised association

d. PDAs are a well-recognised association

e. Diastolic doming is clearly seen in >50% of patients

16 In Marfan's syndrome, the following are true:

a. Is commonly associated with neuromuscular disease

b. Aortic root surgery should be delayed until the root measures 5.5 cm

c. The most common cause of death is aortic dissection

d. Left atrial compression is a recognised complication

e. In the presence of dissection, the true lumen is commonly the smallest

17 In the presence of hypoplastic left heart syndrome, the following features are seen:

a. AS

b. MS

c. Diminutive LV

d. Severe hypoplasia of the ascending aorta

e. Coronary artery perfusion is via the PDA connection

18 With regard to congenital AS, the following are true:
  a. Unicuspid valves are a recognised cause
  b. An acommisural pattern is recognised
  c. A unicommisural pattern is recognised
  d. Annual follow-up is only recommended in adulthood
  e. Doming of the valve is best seen in the parasternal long-axis view at peak systole

19 In Noonan's syndrome, the following features are well recognised:
  a. Tricuspid stenosis
  b. PS
  c. ASDs
  d. Cardiomyopathy
  e. Dilated aorta

20 In Turner's syndrome, the following cardiac anomalies are frequently seen:
  a. Bicuspid AV
  b. Coarctation of the aorta
  c. PDA
  d. Tricuspid dysplasia
  e. PS

Adult Congenital Heart Disease

ANSWERS

1 a. T
  b. F
  c. F
  d. T
  e. F

Ebstein's anomaly causes atrialisation of the RV because the TV is apically displaced causing a large RA. It is not associated with an increased risk of malignancy in later life. There is failure of coaptation leading to significant TR. Tricuspid stenosis is not a feature and at least 50% are associated with an ASD or PFO.

2 a. T
  b. T
  c. T
  d. F
  e. T

In a Fontan's circulation, there is a single ventricle functioning as the systemic ventricle. This is usually a morphological LV, although a morphological RV can sometimes be seen. The pulmonary blood flow comes either directly from the RA or from the IVC depending on the type of surgical repair. Arrhythmias are generally poorly tolerated because LV filling time is reduced and there is no RV to 'pump' blood into the LV. Dehydration is also a problem as pulmonary blood flow (and therefore LV filling) is crucially dependent on high right-sided pressures to drive blood into the PA.

3 a. T
  b. T
  c. F
  d. F
  e. T

In complete transposition of the great arteries there is ventriculo–arterial discordance such that the RV connects to the aorta and the LV to the PA. The pulmonary and systemic circulations are separate unless there is a communication at atrial, ventricular or arterial level. Early surgical corrections involved creating an atrial septostomy to allow mixing of systemic and pulmonary blood at the atrial level. As the two circulations would be unconnected without this, patients would otherwise die soon after birth. A Mustard or Senning operation creates intra-atrial baffles to route blood from the systemic venous return through the septum into the LA and from the pulmonary veins to the RA. With these procedures the morphological RV is the systemic ventricle, but if the patient has had an arterial switch early in life, the morphological LV is the systemic ventricle. The pulmonary veins are not detached as part of surgical correction of transposition. The patient may be cyanosed depending on the presence or otherwise of a VSD, pulmonary hypertension, exercise etc.

4 a. F
  b. T
  c. F
  d. F
  e. F

In congenitally corrected transposition there is both atrioventricular and ventriculo–arterial discordance such that the RA connects to the morphological LV and the LV to the PA. The moderator band is always found in the morphological RV as is the TV. The atrioventricular valves are always attached to the corresponding ventricle, thus the MV is always with the morphological LV. The morphological LV (pulmonic ventricle) gives rise to the PA whereas the morphological RV (systemic ventricle) gives rise to the aorta. The IVC and SVC drain as usual into the RA, which drains into the pulmonic ventricle (i.e. the morphological LV), whereas the pulmonary veins drain as usual into the LA, which drains into the systemic ventricle (i.e. the morphological RV). No VSD is required to provide communication between systemic and pulmonary circulations in order to maintain life as they are not independent.

5 a. T
  b. F
  c. T
  d. T
  e. T

Ostium secundum defects are generally centrally located in the atrial septum and are the commonest type. The subcostal view is the optimal view for detecting ASDs, although other views can be useful. Shunts are generally left to right and therefore right-sided dilatation is seen. Sinus venosus defects are the most peripherally located defects in the atrial septum, close to the entrance of the SVC or IVC and as such, anomalous pulmonary venous drainage is frequently seen. Selected cases of ostium secundum ASDs can be closed percutaneously with closure devices.

6 a. F
  b. T
  c. F
  d. T
  e. T

The shunt is left to right, unless there is severe pulmonary hypertension. The left-to-right shunt here is at the level of the PA, therefore no RA or RV dilatation occurs. Instead, the pulmonary circulation is volume overloaded causing left-sided return to also be volume overloaded leading to left heart dilatation. In diastole, when the AV is closed, aortic blood shunts back through the PDA into to PA; this causes diastolic flow reversal on Doppler in the descending aorta, similar to that seen in AR. The normal function of the PDA in utero is to shunt blood from the PA into the aorta and bypass the lungs, which do not serve any ventilatory function.

7 a. T
  b. T
  c. F
  d. T
  e. T

Perimembranous VSDs are the most common type. Inlet VSDs are high in the ventricular septum and can be associated with other abnormalities in the central fibrous body such as ASDs or AVSDs. With a left-to-right shunting VSD, blood moves in systole from LV to RV to PA without pooling in the RV, therefore RV dilatation does not occur. As with PDAs, increased pulmonary blood flow and therefore pulmonary venous return to the LA causes LA and LV dilatation due to volume overload. A small VSD is restrictive and minimal equalisation of pressures occurs, leading to a high pressure gradient between LV and RV, causing a high velocity Doppler signal on CW. Some perimembranous VSDs close spontaneously leaving a small ventricular septal aneurysm as a remnant.

8 a. T
   b. F
   c. T
   d. T
   e. T

Coarctations are rare but can cause significant hypertension. On CW Doppler, velocities will always be in the forward direction in systole and diastole, though maximal velocity will be in systole. BP in the legs can be lower than that measured in the arms due to restriction of flow from the coarctation. Suprasternal views are not always the clearest depending on the orientation of the aorta and location of the coarctation, so CT or MRI is superior in these situations. Coarctations and bicuspid AVs are associated.

9 a. F
   b. T
   c. F
   d. T
   e. F

The foramen ovale allows the passage of blood from the RA to LA in utero. In adulthood, PFOs can allow transient flow of blood from RA to LA during spontaneous breathing or Valsalva, with the potential for the passage of embolic material into the systemic circulation causing strokes. However, as there is no continuous flow across a PFO (unlike an ASD), there is no equalisation of pressures of RA and LA and there is no associated right heart dilatation. Agitated saline is ideally administered via the femoral vein as the bubbles are more directly delivered onto the atrial septum from the IVC than the SVC (antecubital veins).

10 a. T
   b. T
   c. T
   d. F
   e. T

The PS may be subvalvular, which would cause a high RVOT peak velocity. A dilated PA may be seen with PS causing post-stenotic dilatation. The VSD can shunt either left to right ('pink' tetralogy) or right to left (Eisenmenger's physiology). Hypertrophy of the RV walls is seen, not thinning.

11 a. T
   b. T
   c. T
   d. T
   e. T

The VSD is commonly of the muscular type and the aortic root overrides the ventricular septum, exiting both the RV and LV, because of anterior displacement. Rarely, the LAD coronary artery may arise from the RCA coronary artery. In all types of congenital heart disease with significant left-to-right shunting, the presence of PS provides a degree of protection to the pulmonary vasculature from developing pulmonary hypertension. Numerous surgical shunts have been used historically to palliate Tetralogy of Fallot of which the Blalock–Taussig shunt is one.

12 a. T
   b. T
   c. F
   d. T
   e. T

All are correct except the Blalock–Taussig shunt connects the subclavian artery to the PA.

13 a. T
   b. T
   c. T
   d. F
   e. F

The Rastelli procedure utilises a manufactured graft to close the VSD and direct left ventricular blood to the aorta. An artificial conduit is then created to direct deoxygenated blood from the RV to a reconstructed main PA bifurcation. The Fontan circulation usually connects the RA to the PA allowing the single ventricle to function as the systemic ventricle. The Norwood procedure connects the main PA to the ascending aorta. Blood therefore exits the ventricle through the PV into the aorta; mixing of oxygenated and deoxygenated blood is created via a Blalock–Taussig shunt. The Damus–Kaye–Stansel is a similar procedure where the proximal PA is connected to the ascending aorta in the double-inlet LV with subaortic stenosis. The Konno procedure is a AVR with widening of the aortic root and ascending aorta in patients with subaortic stenosis and hypoplasia of the aortic outflow tract.

14 a. F
   b. T
   c. F
   d. T
   e. T

The PA pressure cannot be calculated from the data given. A TR (or PR) jet velocity would be required to accurately gauge this; the step-up in velocity across the RVOT is suggestive of mild PS. A volume overloaded right heart is in keeping with an ASD; a VSD usually causes left heart rather than right heart dilatation. The $Q_p:Q_s$ shunt is given by the ratio of SVs (CSA × VTI) across the RVOT and LVOT, which calculates at around 3.5:1.

15 a. T
   b. F
   c. T
   d. T
   e. F

Familial screening for bicuspid valves is now recommended under the latest ACC/AHA guidelines, as it is recognised as an inherited congenital anomaly. Prolapse is seen in >80% of patients. VSDs and PDAs are recognised conditions that coexist with a bicuspid AV. The presence of *systolic* doming is seen in >50% of patients.

16 a. F
   b. F
   c. T
   d. T
   e. T

Marfan's syndrome is a connective tissue disease. The decision for surgical intervention should be considered at a root measurement of 4.5 cm. The most common cause of death is due to aortic dissection, and LA compression is a well-recognised complication due to the size of the dilatation. The true lumen within the aortic dissection is commonly the smaller of the two lumens.

17 a. T
   b. T

c. T

d. T

e. T

Hypoplastic left heart syndrome is thought to result from premature closure of the foramen ovale in utero leading to an underdeveloped LV and its inflow and outflow components. There is a spectrum of severity that can include any or all of the complications mentioned.

18 a. T

   b. T

   c. T

   d. F

   e. T

Unicuspid valves are well recognised and can be of the rare acommissural type or the more common unicommissural type. AS can present at any stage from infancy, sometimes being delayed because of the co-presence of AR. Follow-up should therefore reflect this. Although the number of cusps is best seen in the short-axis view, doming is best demonstrated in the long-axis view.

19 a. F

   b. T

   c. T

   d. T

   e. F

Noonan's syndrome is associated with PS, ASD and cardiomyopathy.

20 a. T

   b. T

   c. F

   d. F

   e. F

In Turner's syndrome, the AV and root are mainly involved, with bicuspid valves/aortic coarctation being seen in approximately 10–15% of patients. Other abnormalities can include partial anomalous pulmonary venous drainage.

9 Video Questions

CASE 1

VIDEOS 1.1, 1.2, 1.3, 1.4, 1.5, 1.6, 1.7

Questions

A 28-year-old man attends his local cardiology department for annual follow-up. He is asymptomatic. His echo is shown.

Case Figure 1.1

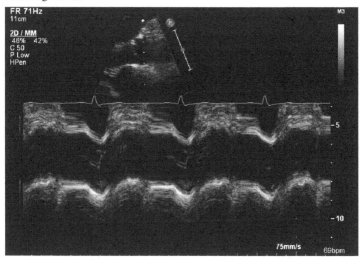

Successful Accreditation in Echocardiography: A Self-Assessment Guide,
First Edition. Sanjay M. Banypersad and Keith Pearce.
© 2012 John Wiley & Sons, Ltd. Published 2012 by John Wiley & Sons, Ltd.

Case Figure 1.2

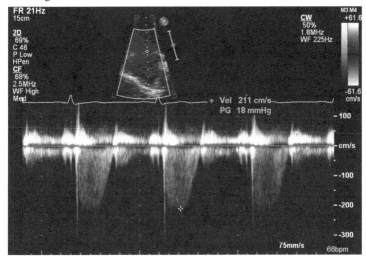

Case Figure 1.3

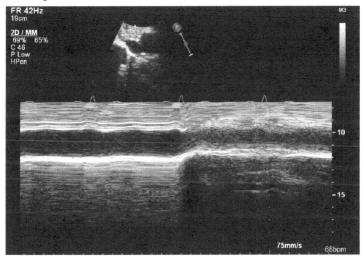

Select ONE option only for each of the questions below.

1 With regard to the atria:
  a. An LA myxoma is present
  b. Cor triatriatum is seen
  c. An ASD occluder device is present
  d. An RA thrombus is present
  e. A PFO with thrombus is seen

2 Which of the following statements is true regarding the estimated RA pressure:
   a. RA pressure is negligible
   b. RA pressure is approximately 10 mmHg
   c. RA pressure is likely >20 mmHg
   d. RA pressure cannot be estimated from the data
   e. Hepatic vein size is not affected by RA pressure

3 With regard to the original cardiac pathology in this case:
   a. Flow across the septum is only seen on valsalva
   b. Right to left flow is most commonly expected
   c. RA myxomas are more common than LA myxomas
   d. These defects can be closed percutaneously
   e. Thrombus crossing an ASD is not recognised

4 Which of the following statements is false:
   a. The RA is dilated
   b. The RV is dilated
   c. LV function is normal
   d. Pulmonary hypertension is not present
   e. Paradoxical septal motion is seen

Video Questions

CASE 2

VIDEOS 2.1, 2.2, 2.3, 2.4, 2.5, 2.6, 2.7

Questions

An 80-year-old lady presents with weight loss and haemoptysis. She is a current smoker. Her echo is shown.

Case Figure 2.1

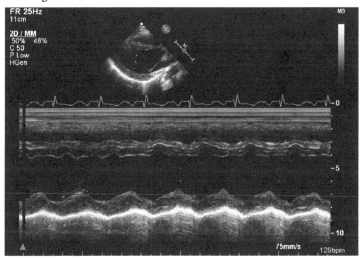

Select ONE option only for each of the questions below.

1 The following is true regarding the mass:
   a. It is artefactual, as it is not present in all views
   b. Embolisation into the systemic circulation is very likely
   c. Myocardial contrast enhancement imaging has been performed to try and demonstrate vascularity
   d. It is most likely a vegetation
   e. None of the above

2 With regards to the pericardial effusion:
   a. It is trivial in size
   b. Appears localised around the RV
   c. Appears global
   d. It is large
   e. Appears localised around the LV

3 The M-mode image shows:
   a. Dilated LV cavity
   b. Paradoxical septal motion
   c. Early MV closure
   d. Mass in the LA
   e. None of the above

4 The most likely diagnosis is:
   a. Tumour
   b. Thrombus
   c. Vegetation
   d. Artefact
   e. ARVC

Video Questions

CASE 3

VIDEOS 3.1, 3.2, 3.3, 3.4, 3.5, 3.6, 3.7,
3.8, 3.9, 3.10, 3.11

Questions

This echo is of a 23-year-old woman who was found to have a soft systolic murmur on auscultation. She has no symptoms and her ECG is normal.

Case Figure 3.1

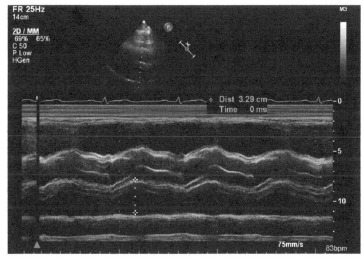

Case Figure 3.2

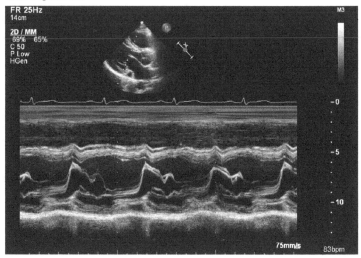

Case Figure 3.3

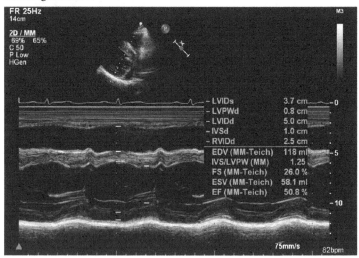

Case Figure 3.4

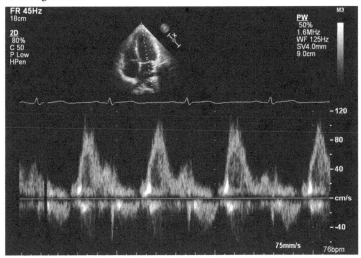

Select ONE option only for each of the questions below.

1 The mitral Doppler inflow suggests:
   a. Normal transmitral flow
   b. Impaired LV relaxation
   c. Pseudonormalisation
   d. Severe diastolic dysfunction
   e. None of the above

2 Which of the following statements are true:
   a. IVC collapse is normal
   b. Mild AR is present
   c. LV function is moderately impaired
   d. Subcostal colour flow suggests an ASD is present
   e. None of the above

3 With regard to the abnormality seen in the parasternal long-axis view, the likely diagnosis is:
   a. An abscess
   b. An angiosarcoma
   c. A pericardial cyst causing extrinsic compression of the LA
   d. A coronary artery aneurysm
   e. A dilated coronary sinus

4 The following statements is false:

    a. The AV is tricuspid

    b. A persistent left-sided SVC could explain the echo findings

    c. Injection of the agitated saline into the left arm will help establish the diagnosis

    d. Injection of agitated saline into the right arm with valsalva manoeuvre will help establish the diagnosis

    e. RV function is normal

Video Questions

CASE 4

VIDEOS 4.1, 4.2, 4.3, 4.4, 4.5, 4.6, 4.7, 4.8, 4.9, 4.10

Questions

A hypertensive 65-year-old woman has an echo because of a diastolic murmur on auscultation. The echo is shown.

Case Figure 4.1

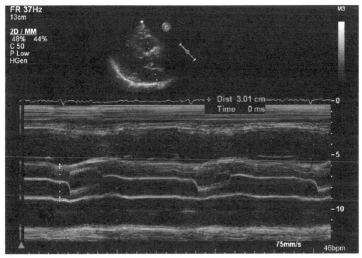

Case Figure 4.2

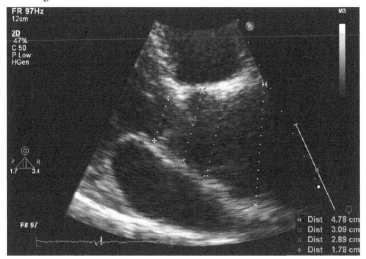

Case Figure 4.3

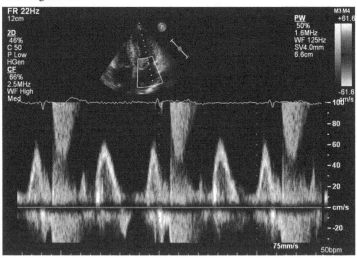

Case Figure 4.4

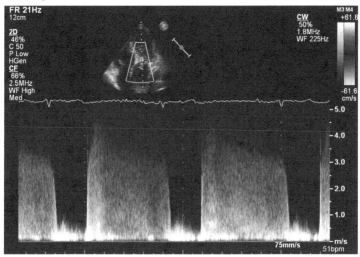

Case Figure 4.5

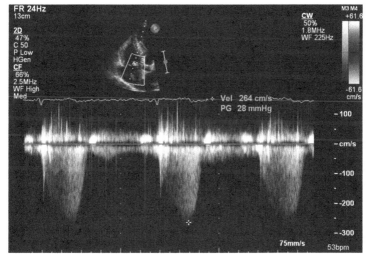

Select ONE option only for each of the questions below.

1 The degree of AR is:
   a. There is no AR
   b. Mild
   c. Moderate
   d. Severe
   e. Torrential

2 Which of the following statements is false:
   a. The ascending aorta is dilated
   b. The arch is dilated
   c. The descending aorta is dilated
   d. There is symmetrical LVH
   e. The TR is mild

3 Which of the following statements is false:
   a. Overall, LV systolic function is good
   b. The AR could be secondary to hypertension
   c. The aortic dilatation could be secondary to Marfan's syndrome
   d. If the diagnosis of Marfan's is made, aortic surgery is not indicated
   e. The conformation of the aortic root sinuses can be lost in Ehlers–Danlos syndrome

4 The following is true of the LVOT/aortic root in this echo:
   a. It is prosthetic
   b. The sinus of valsalva is dilated
   c. The sinotubular junction is dilated
   d. There is evidence of systolic anterior motion of the MV chorda into the LVOT
   e. None of the above

Video Questions

CASE 5

> **VIDEOS 5.1, 5.2, 5.3, 5.4, 5.5, 5.6, 5.7, 5.8, 5.9, 5.10, 5.11**

Questions

A 35-year-old woman presents with worsening exertional dyspnoea over 3 months following a viral illness. She has no chest pain. She is a non-smoker. ECG shows LBBB. The basal septum thickness is 0.5 cm and the LV is 6 cm at end-diastole. Peak LVOT velocity is 0.8 m/s and peak aortic velocity is 1.2 m/s.

Case Figure 5.1

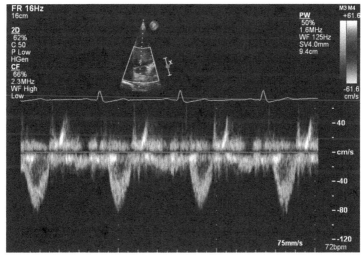

Case Figure 5.2

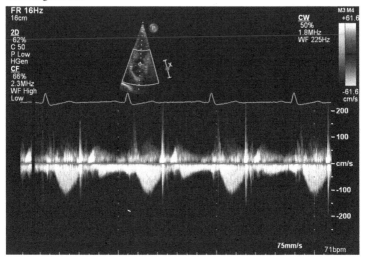

Select ONE option only for each of the questions below.

1 The following best describe the LV **except**:
   a. Dilated
   b. At least moderately impaired
   c. Global reduction in function
   d. Intra-cavity obliteration
   e. None of the above

2 Which of the following are potential causes of this appearance:
   a. Myocarditis
   b. Dilated cardiomyopathy
   c. Uninfarcted, hibernating myocardium due to coronary artery disease
   d. End-stage RCM
   e. All of the above

3 Which of the following statements is true regarding the AV in this study:
   a. Normal
   b. Mild AS
   c. Mild AR
   d. Mixed AV disease
   e. Bicuspid AV

4 The following best describes the MV in this study:
  a. Severely thickened and calcified
  b. Calcified annulus with moderate MS
  c. Thin and mobile leaflets
  d. Mild MR
  e. Ruptured chordae

Video Questions

CASE 6

> **VIDEOS 6.1, 6.2, 6.3, 6.4, 6.5, 6.6, 6.7, 6.8, 6.9, 6.10**

Questions

A 30-year-old woman who is normally fit and well presents with palpitations. Here ECG reveals an accessory pathway.

Case Figure 6.1

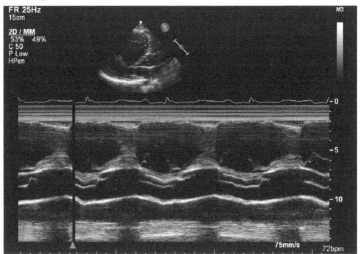

Case Figure 6.2

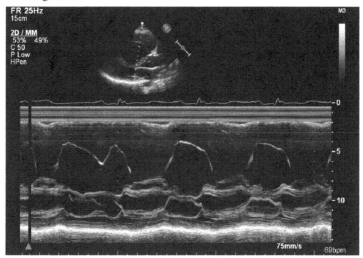

Case Figure 6.3

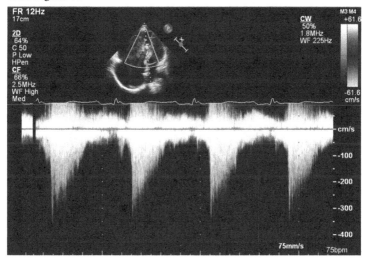

Select ONE option only for each of the questions below.

1 The most likely diagnosis is:
   a. Isolated LV non-compaction
   b. Tetralogy of Fallot
   c. Cor triatriatum
   d. Ebstein's anomaly
   e. Double-outlet LV

2 Which of the following statements best describes the TR:
   a. At least moderate, eccentric TR directed along the septum
   b. Central, functional, severe TR
   c. Severe central TR directed along the septum
   d. Mild–moderate, functional TR
   e. Mild, eccentric TR directed along the septum

3 Which of the following statements is **not** true:
   a. There is paradoxical septal motion
   b. A Eustachian valve is seen
   c. There is mild MR
   d. The RA is significantly dilated
   e. All of the above

4 The following are associated with this condition:
   a. Anomalous pulmonary venous drainage
   b. Arrhythmias
   c. ASD
   d. PFO
   e. All of the above

Video Questions

CASE 7

VIDEOS 7.1, 7.2, 7.3, 7.4, 7.5, 7.6, 7.7,
7.8, 7.9, 7.10, 7.11, 7.12

Questions

A 55-year-old man presents with worsening shortness of breath on exertion. His BP is normal but his ECG is abnormal with voltage criteria for LVH. His echo is shown. 2D measurements reveal IVSd 1.8 cm, PW 1.8 cm, LVEDD 5.5 cm.

Case Figure 7.1

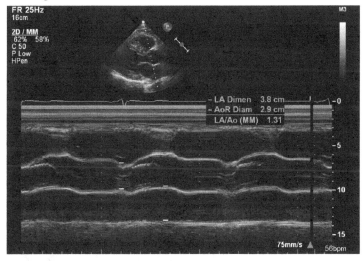

Case Figure 7.2

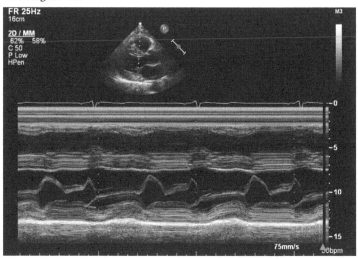

Case Figure 7.3

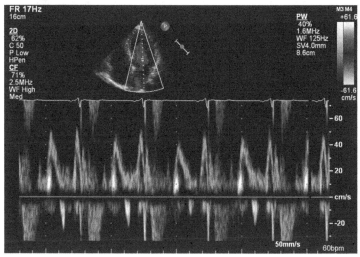

Case Figure 7.4

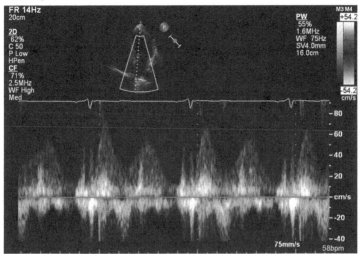

Case Figure 7.5

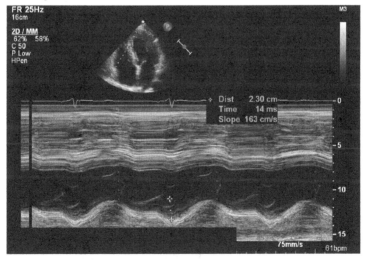

Case Figure 7.6

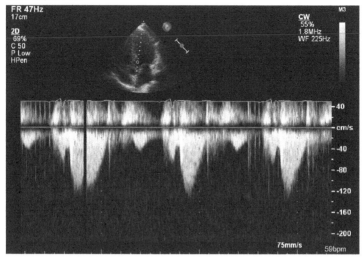

Case Figure 7.7

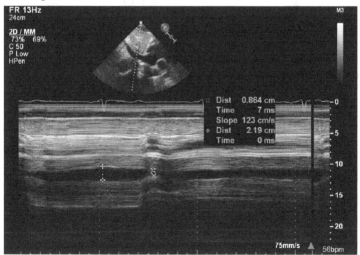

Select ONE option only for each of the questions below.

1 The following best describes the LVH:
   a. Moderate, asymmetrical affecting predominantly posterior wall
   b. Moderate, symmetrical
   c. Severe, asymmetrical affecting predominantly the septum
   d. Severe, symmetrical
   e. Severe, asymmetrical affecting predominantly the posterior wall

2 The following statements are true **except**:
   a. TAPSE suggests mildly impaired RV function
   b. In the context of LVH, the transmitral Doppler may represent abnormal diastology
   c. Loss of longitudinal contraction is apparent in the apical 4-chamber view
   d. The LV is of normal size
   e. There is no evidence of LVOT obstruction due to the LVH

3 Which of the following statements are true:
   a. IVC collapses by 75% on sniffing
   b. The IVC is not dilated
   c. There is mild MR
   d. There is no AR or TR
   e. All of the above

4 Which of the following is the **least** likely diagnosis:
   a. Ischaemic heart disease
   b. Fabry's disease
   c. Hypertrophic cardiomyopathy
   d. Infiltrative cardiomyopathy
   e. Amyloidosis

Video Questions

CASE 8

VIDEOS 8.1, 8.2, 8.3, 8.4, 8.5, 8.6, 8.7, 8.8, 8.9

Questions

A 40-year-old woman presents with palpitations. Her ECG is normal but she has a systolic murmur on auscultation. She has the echo shown.

Case Figure 8.1

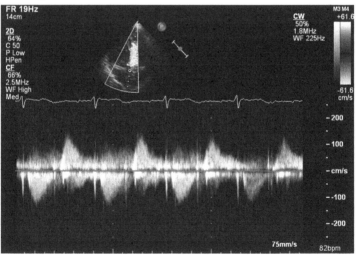

Case Figure 8.2

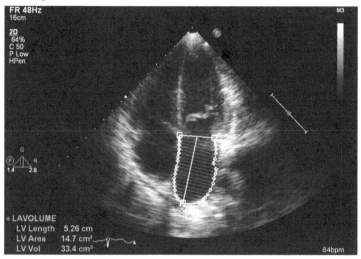

Case Figure 8.3

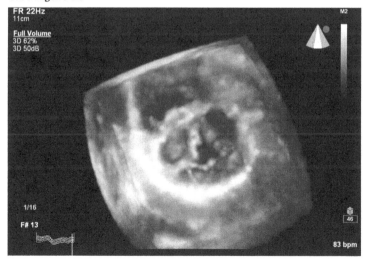

Select ONE option only for each of the questions below.

1 The following best describes the MR:
   a. Severe, central MR with systolic flow reversal in the pulmonary veins
   b. Severe, eccentric MR, directed posteriorly
   c. Moderate central MR with systolic flow reversal in the pulmonary veins
   d. Severe eccentric MR, directed anteriorly
   e. Mild, eccentric MR directed posteriorly

2 The aetiology of the MR is:
   a. Leaflet prolapse
   b. Leaflet tethering
   c. Functional
   d. Ischaemic
   e. None of the above

3 The following is also seen:
   a. Bicuspid AV
   b. Mild TR
   c. Increased LA volumes
   d. Ruptured MV chordae
   e. Severely impaired LV with annular dilatation

4 The 3D image confirms:
   a. Commissural fusion of the anterior MV leaflet
   b. Malcoaptation of the leaflets
   c. Cleft anterior MV leaflet
   d. P2 prolapse of the posterior MV leaflet
   e. None of the above

Video Questions

CASE 9

VIDEOS 9.1, 9.2, 9.3, 9.4, 9.5, 9.6, 9.7

Questions

A 68-year-old woman with diabetes, hypertension and high cholesterol presents with a stroke. Her echo is shown.

Case Figure 9.1

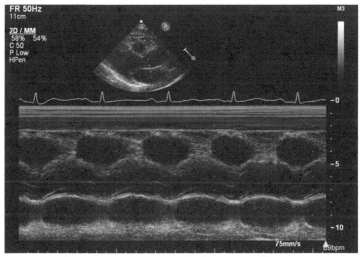

Case Figure 9.2

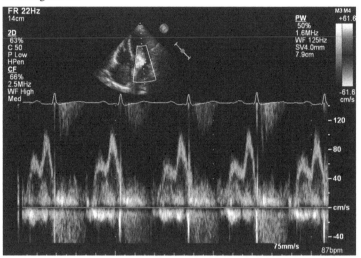

Case Figure 9.3

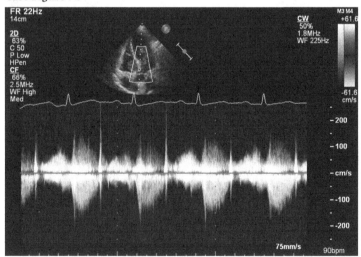

Case Figure 9.4

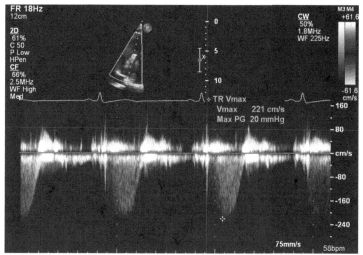

Select ONE option only for each of the questions below.

1 The transmitral E and A velocities:
   a. May be normal for the patient's age
   b. Indicate severe diastolic dysfunction
   c. Indicate the presence of MS
   d. Indicate anomalous pulmonary venous drainage
   e. Are not affected by the presence of severe MR

2 Which of the following best describes the TR in this study:
   a. There is no TR
   b. Mild–moderate
   c. Moderate–severe
   d. Severe
   e. Free (torrential)

3 The following best describes the mass:
   a. It is attached to the atrial septum by a stalk
   b. It may be attached to the TV
   c. Straddles a PFO into the LA
   d. It is fluid filled
   e. It is vascular

4 The following statements are true:

   a. The mass is responsible for the stroke

   b. The AV is bicuspid

   c. LV function is impaired

   d. There is a small global pericardial effusion

   e. None of the above

Video Questions

CASE 10

> **VIDEOS 10.1, 10.2, 10.3, 10.4, 10.5, 10.6, 10.7**

Questions

A 73-year-old man presents with fever for a few weeks. His blood cultures are positive for *Streptococcus Viridans* and he is commenced on empirical IV antibiotics. After 1 week he suffers a stroke. An echo is performed shortly after.

Case Figure 10.1

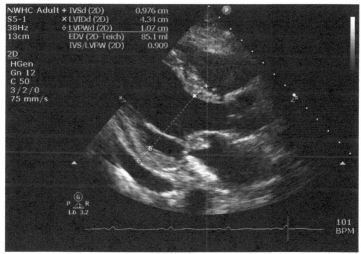

Case Figure 10.2

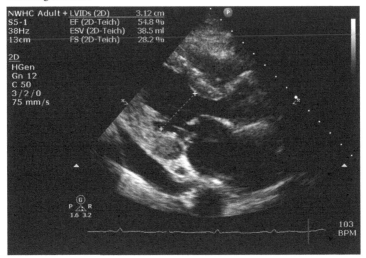

Case Figure 10.3

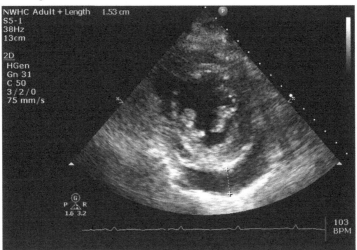

Select ONE option only for each of the questions below.

1 The pericardial effusion is:
   a. Small
   b. Moderate with no significant haemodynamic compromise
   c. Moderate with significant haemodynamic compromise
   d. Large with no significant haemodynamic compromise
   e. Large with significant haemodynamic compromise

2 The primary abnormality is:
   a. Vegetation attached to anterior leaflet with posteriorly directed MR
   b. Vegetation attached to anterior leaflet with anteriorly directed MR
   c. Vegetation attached to posterior leaflet with posteriorly directed MR
   d. Vegetation attached to posterior leaflet with anteriorly directed MR
   e. Vegetations attached to both leaflets with anteriorly directed MR

3 The diagnosis of endocarditis with acute, severe MR is made. The EF of 55% (by 2D measurements) suggests the LV systolic function in this situation is:
   a. Normal
   b. Hyperdynamic
   c. Mild–moderately impaired
   d. Moderate–severely impaired
   e. Severely impaired

4 Which of the following statements is **false**:
   a. A TOE may be useful to rule out an aortic root abscess
   b. The vegetation may be implicated in the man's stroke
   c. Surgery should be considered
   d. Blood cultures do not form part of the Duke's criteria
   e. New valvular regurgitation is one of the Duke's criteria

Video Questions

CASE 11

> **VIDEOS 11.1, 11.2, 11.3, 11.4, 11.5, 11.6, 11.7, 11.8, 11.9, 11.10, 11.11, 11.12**

Questions

A 53-year-old man presents with worsening ankle oedema. His Chest x-ray shows a large heart and his ECG is normal apart from low QRS voltages. His echo is shown. IVSd 2.1 cm, LVEDD 4.5 cm, PW 2 cm.

Case Figure 11.1

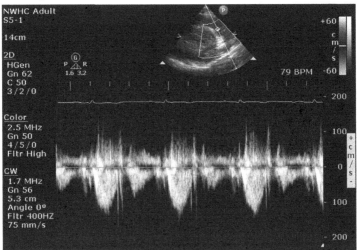

Case Figure 11.2

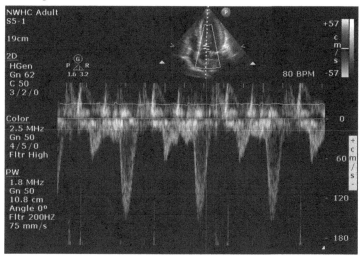

Case Figure 11.3

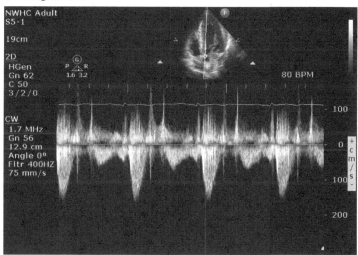

Case Figure 11.4

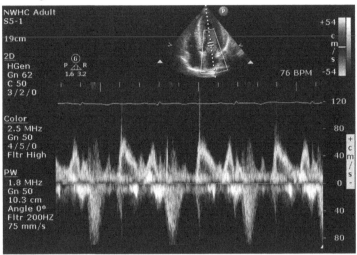

Case Figure 11.5

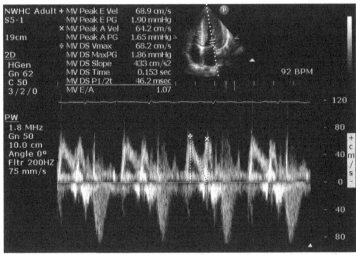

Case Figure 11.6

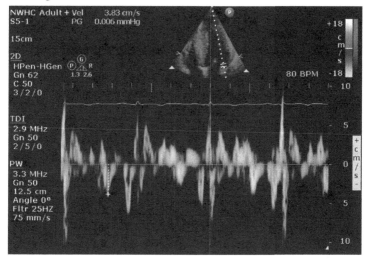

Select ONE option only for each of the questions below.

1 The LVH severity is:
   a. None
   b. Mild
   c. Moderate
   d. Severe

2 The MR severity is?
   a. Severe
   b. Minimal
   c. Moderate
   d. None of the above

3 Which of the following statements is true regarding this study:
   a. There is RVH
   b. Longitudinal contraction is markedly decreased compared
      with radial contraction
   c. The valves appear thickened
   d. All of the above

4 From the lateral wall E:E' provided, the assessment of LV diastolic function is?

    a. Not available

    b. Abnormal

    c. Normal

    d. Unreliable in this setting

5 What is the likeliest diagnosis?

    a. HOCM

    b. Hypertrophic Non-Obstructive Cardiomyopathy

    c. Cardiac amyloidosis

    d. Non-compaction syndrome

Video Questions

CASE 12

VIDEOS 12.1, 12.2, 12.3, 12.4, 12.5, 12.6, 12.7, 12.8

Questions

A 43-year-old woman with a past history of rheumatic fever, presents with exertional dyspnoea over a few months. Her echo is shown.

Case Figure 12.1

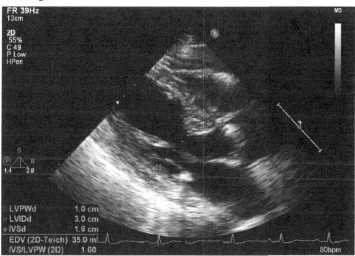

Case Figure 12.2

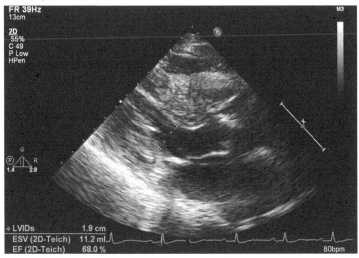

Case Figure 12.3

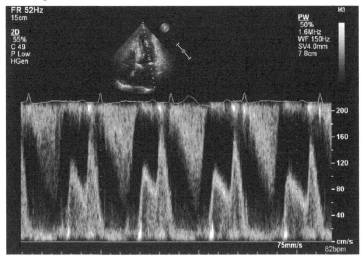

Case Figure 12.4

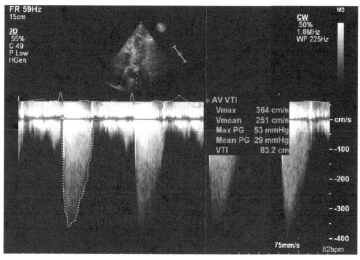

Case Figure 12.5

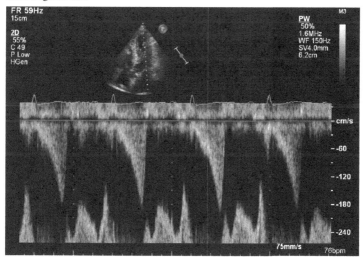

Select ONE option only for each of the questions below.

1 The LV function is?
  a. Globally mildly reduced
  b. Normal
  c. Moderately reduced with inferior hypokinesia
  d. Hyperdynamic

2 The AV CW Doppler VTI suggests:
  a. Mild AS
  b. Moderate AS
  c. Severe AS
  d. None of the above

3 The RV function is?
  a. Normal
  b. Mildly impaired
  c. Moderately impaired
  d. Unable to comment

4 The best fit diagnosis in this case?
  a. AS
  b. Intra-cavity obliteration
  c. Hypertrophic Non-obstructive cardiomyopathy
  d. AS with LVH and intra-cavity obliteration

5 The intra-cavity gradient is best demonstrated by:
  a. Colour Doppler
  b. 2D
  c. CW Doppler
  d. PW Doppler

Video Questions

CASE 13

VIDEOS 13.1, 13.2, 13.3, 13.4, 13.5, 13.6, 13.7, 13.8, 13.9, 13.10

Questions

A 66-year-old woman presents with worsening exertional dyspnoea and peripheral oedema. A preliminary clinical diagnosis of heart failure is made. Her echo is shown.

Case Figure 13.1

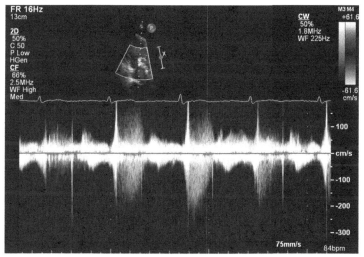

Case Figure 13.2

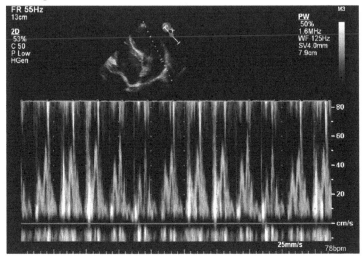

Select ONE option only for each of the questions below.

1 The transmitral Doppler waveform variation with breathing suggests:
   a. <25% decrease with inspiration
   b. <25% decrease with expiration
   c. >25% decrease with inspiration
   d. >25% decrease with expiration
   e. None of the above

2 The extracardiac structure seen in the modified apical 4-chamber view adjacent to the left heart is most likely:
   a. Tumour
   b. Collapsed lung secondary to pleural effusion
   c. Rib
   d. Pericardial drain
   e. Artefact

3 The RV function appears
   a. Normal
   b. Moderately reduced
   c. Severely reduced
   d. Hyperdynamic
   e. Unable to comment

4 Which statement best describes all the salient features?
  a. Global pericardial effusion with RV compromise
  b. Loculated pericardial effusion
  c. Bilateral pleural effusions with small pericardial collection
  d. Posterior pericardial collection only with right heart compromise
  e. Bilateral pleural effusions with no pericardial effusion

Video Questions

CASE 14

VIDEOS 14.1, 14.2, 14.3, 14.4, 14.5, 14.6, 14.7, 14.8, 14.9

Questions

An 80-year-old man presents with exertional syncope. He has suffered worsening chest pain and breathlessness on exertion for some months prior to attending. His echo is shown.

Case Figure 14.1

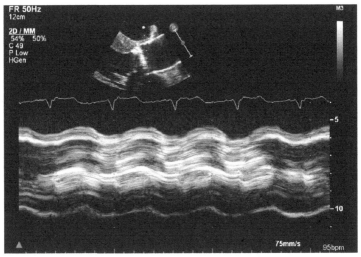

Case Figure 14.2

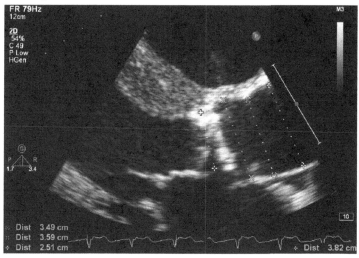

Case Figure 14.3

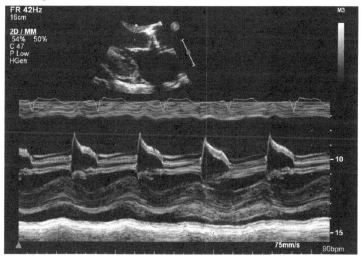

Case Figure 14.4

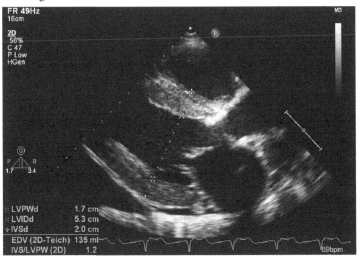

Case Figure 14.5

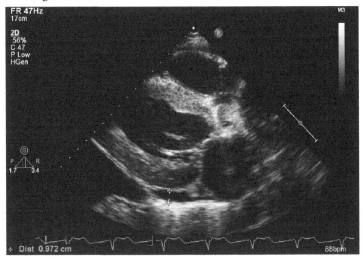

Case Figure 14.6

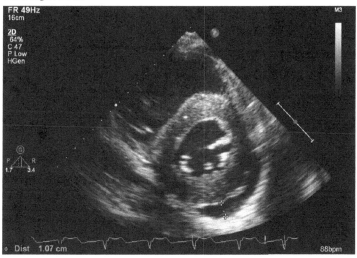

Case Figure 14.7

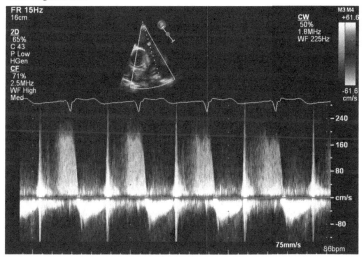

Case Figure 14.8

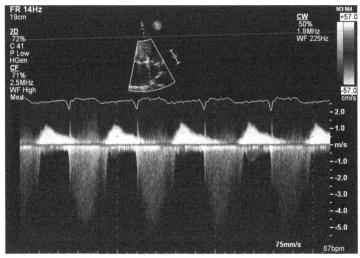

Case Figure 14.9

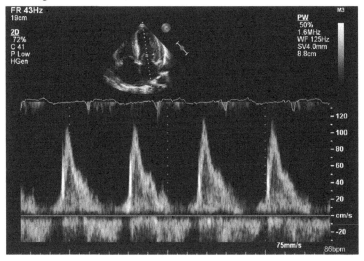

Case Figure 14.10

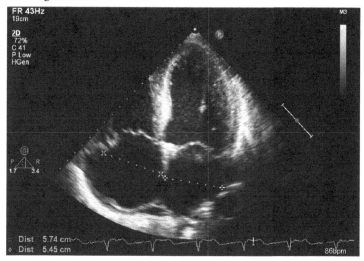

Case Figure 14.11

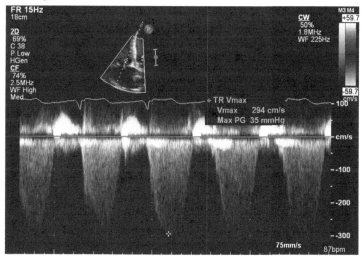

Case Figure 14.12

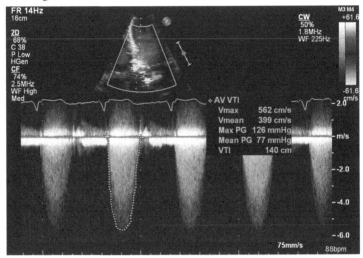

Case Figure 14.13

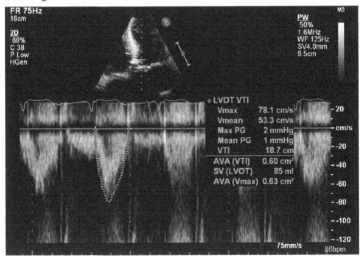

Case Figure 14.14

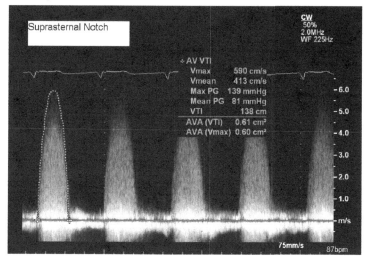

Select ONE option only for each of the questions below.

1 How would you best describe the LV function?
  a. Normal
  b. Mildly impaired with RWMA
  c. Moderate global reduction
  d. Severe global reduction

2 What is the severity of MR
  a. Mild MR
  b. None
  c. Unable to estimate
  d. Moderate MR

3 The LVH is?
  a. Asymmetrical LVH
  b. Mild symmetrical LVH
  c. None
  d. Moderate symmetrical LVH

4 The pericardial collection is
  a. Small posterior non-compromising
  b. Moderate posterior with no RV compromise
  c. Small posterior with RV compromise
  d. Small global with no RV compromise

5 The severity of AS is **best** demonstrated in this situation by:
   a. M-Mode
   b. 2-D echo
   c. AV pressure drop
   d. Continuity equation

Video Questions

CASE 15

VIDEOS 15.1, 15.2, 15.3, 15.4, 15.5, 15.6, 15.7, 15.8, 15.9, 15.10, 15.11, 15.12, 15.13, 15.14, 15.15

Questions

A 63-year-old man presents with worsening breathlessness over 4 weeks culminating in his admission with pulmonary oedema. His echo is shown.

Case Figure 15.1

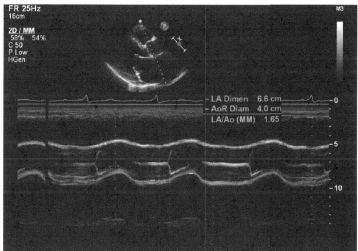

Case Figure 15.2

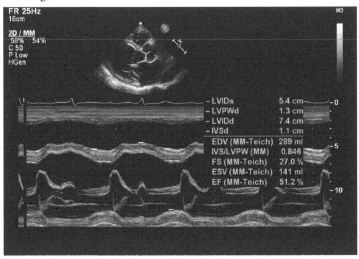

Case Figure 15.3

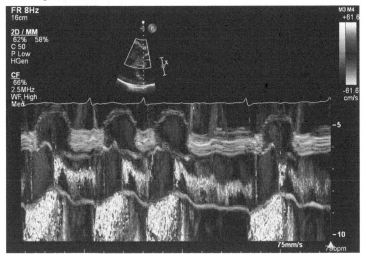

Case Figure 15.4

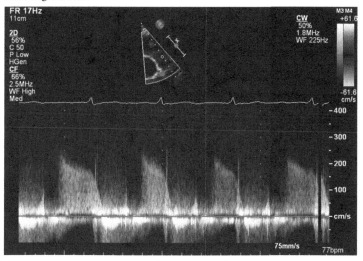

Case Figure 15.5

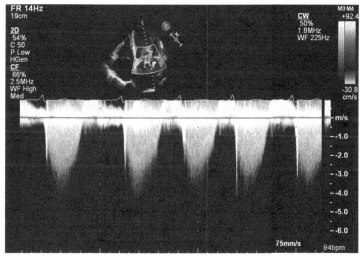

Case Figure 15.6

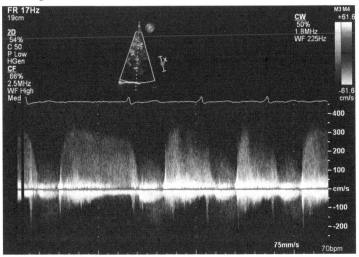

Case Figure 15.7

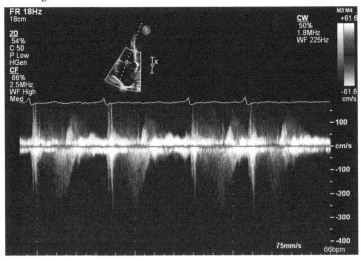

Case Figure 15.8

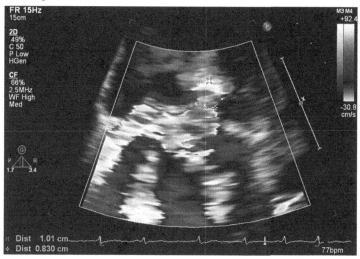

Case Figure 15.9

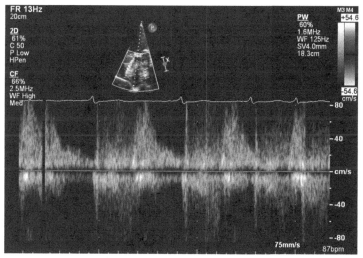

Case Figure 15.10

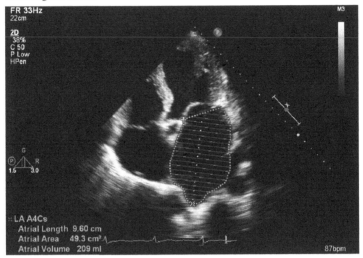

Select ONE option only for each of the questions below.

1 The following are seen in this study:
   a. Mild TR
   b. Mild AR
   c. Mild PR
   d. All of the above

2 Which of the following methods of assessing severity of MR are demonstrated:
   a. Vena contracta
   b. PISA
   c. LA volume
   d. All of the above

3 Which of the following statements are **false:**
   a. The LV is dilated
   b. The colour M-mode shows >60% LVOT width of AR
   c. The estimated MR regurgitant orifice area cannot be calculated from the data provided
   d. The MR is severe and eccentric

4 Which of the following most accurately quantifies the severity of the MR in this situation:

a. MR regurgitant fraction

b. Vena contracta

c. Pulmonary venous Doppler

d. MR regurgitant volume

5 The aetiology of the MR is:

a. A2 prolapse

b. P2 prolapse

c. Tethered posterior leaflet

d. Posterior leaflet perforation

Video Questions

CASE 16

VIDEOS 16.1, 16.2, 16.3, 16.4, 16.5,
16.6, 16.7, 16.8, 16.9, 16.10

Questions

A 60-year-old man who drinks alcohol to excess presents with worsening heart failure symptoms. He is breathless on minimal exertion. His ECG shows LBBB. His angiogram shows normal coronary arteries. His echo is shown.

Case Figure 16.1

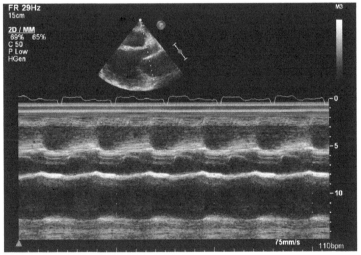

Case Figure 16.2

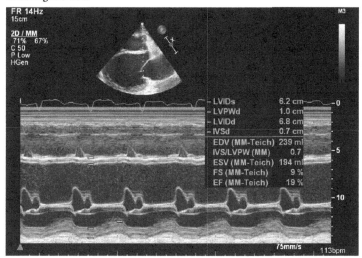

Case Figure 16.3

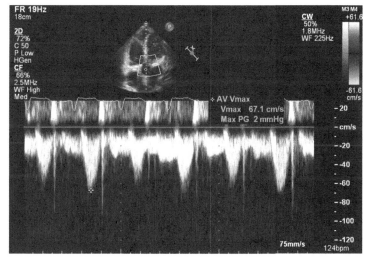

Case Figure 16.4

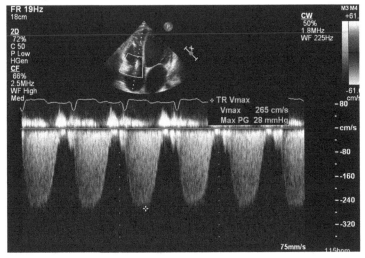

Select ONE option only for each of the questions below.

1 How would you best describe the LV?
   a. RWMAs
   b. Moderate global dysfunction
   c. Dilated LV cavity with severely reduced function
   d. Normal size cavity with a severe reduction in function

2 What is the PA pressure likely to be?
   a. <30 mmHg
   b. 30–40 mmHg
   c. 40–50 mmHg
   d. Unable to estimate from images given

3 The likely diagnosis is:
   a. LV non-compaction syndrome
   b. Early-stage RCM
   c. Pulmonary embolus
   d. Non-ischaemic dilated cardiomyopathy

4 What treatment option should be considered?
   a. Biventricular pacing
   b. Coronary artery bypass grafting
   c. Percutaneous transluminal coronary angioplasty
   d. MVR

5 The most likely aetiology of the MR is:
   a. Ischaemic
   b. Functional due to annular dilatation
   c. MVP
   d. Anterior leaflet perforation

Video Questions

CASE 17

VIDEOS 17.1, 17.2, 17.3, 17.4, 17.5, 17.6, 17.7, 17.8, 17.9, 17.10

Questions

A 22-year-old man presents with worsening shortness of breath on exertion. His past medical history reveals that he has had a dental extraction for a tooth abscess 4 months previously, and recalls feeling flu-like symptoms for 2–3 weeks afterwards but did not seek medical attention. His blood tests, including inflammatory markers, are normal.

Case Figure 17.1

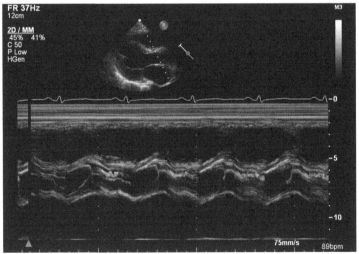

Case Figure 17.2

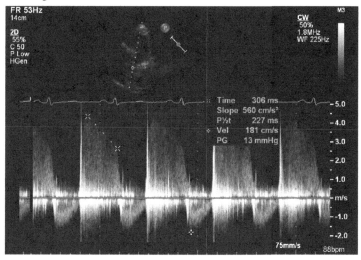

Case Figure 17.3

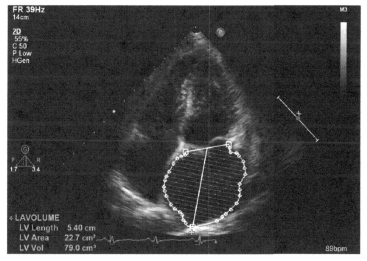

Select ONE option only for each of the questions below.

1 From the images provided, which feature best demonstrates the severity of AR:
   a. Diastolic flow reversal in aortic arch
   b. Colour Doppler signal
   c. AR pressure half time
   d. Hyperdynamic LV function

2 From the data given the AR is:
   a. None
   b. Mild
   c. Moderate
   d. Severe

3 The LV systolic function is?
   a. Normal–hyperdynamic
   b. Mildly reduced with inferior RWMA
   c. Mildly reduced with anterior RWMA
   d. Moderately global reduction

4 In the parasternal long-axis view, the following is true of the AV:
   a. Nodules of Arantius are seen
   b. There is a mobile mass attached to it
   c. The apparent mass is artefactual
   d. Lambl's excrescences are seen

5 What is the likely aetiology of the AR
   a. Valve leaflet prolapse
   b. Endocarditis
   c. Papillary fibroelastoma
   d. Dilated annulus

Video Questions

CASE 18

VIDEOS 18.1, 18.2, 18.3, 18.4, 18.5, 18.6, 18.7

Questions

CASE 18:

A 17-year-old girl who is normally fit and well presents with a few months of worsening ankle oedema and chest pain on exertion. There is no significant past medical history.

Case Figure 18.1

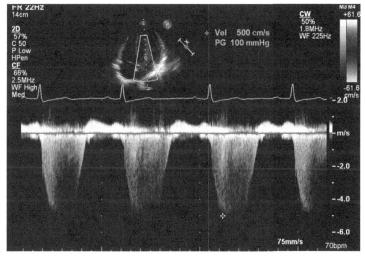

Select ONE option only for each of the questions below.

1 Which of the following is **not** seen:
   a. The RV is the systemic ventricle
   b. The pulmonary veins drain into the LA
   c. The PA is seen exiting the morphological RV
   d. Moderator band

2 Which of the following describes the valves:
   a. The TV opening allows blood flow from the LA into the morphological RV
   b. The TV opening allows blood flow from the RA into the morphological LV
   c. The TV opening allows blood flow from the LA into the morphological LV
   d. The TV opening allows blood flow from the RA into the morphological RV

3 The following best describes the MR:
   a. None
   b. Mild
   c. Moderate
   d. Severe

4 The following is also seen:
   a. Bifurcation of PA into left and right main PA
   b. Normal IVC collapse with respiration
   c. Impaired systemic ventricular function
   d. All of the above

5 The diagnosis is:
   a. Tetralogy of Fallot
   b. Double-outlet LV
   c. Surgically corrected transposition of the great arteries
   d. Congenitally corrected transposition of the great arteries

Video Questions

CASE 19

VIDEOS 19.1, 19.2, 19.3, 19.4, 19.5,
19.6, 19.7, 19.8, 19.9, 19.10

Questions

A 40-year-old man who has had a previous AVR 10 years ago and PPM insertion following complete heart block post-operatively. He had a pacemaker upgrade to a CRT device a year ago. He now re-presents with severe shortness of breath and has been referred for assessment for LVAD implantation. His echo is shown.

Case Figure 19.1

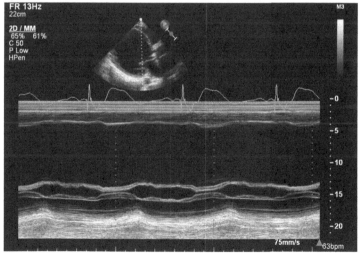

Case Figure 19.2

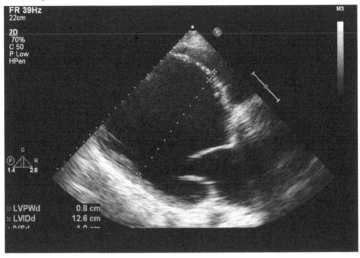

Case Figure 19.3

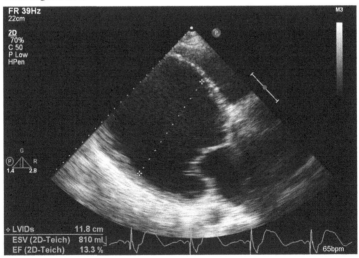

Case Figure 19.4

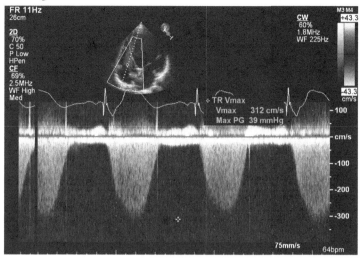

Case Figure 19.5

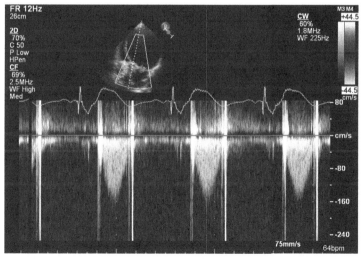

Select ONE option only for each of the questions below.

1 The probable cause of the TR is:
   a. Tricuspid annular dilatation
   b. AVSD
   c. Pacing lead
   d. TV prolapse

2 The following best describes the LV in the parasternal short-axis view:
   a. Severe impairment with global hypokinesia
   b. Severe impairment with postero-lateral hypokinesia
   c. Severe impairment with antero-lateral hypokinesia
   d. Severe LV dilatation with globally severely reduced function

3 What type of contrast agent is used in this case:
   a. Agitated saline
   b. Gelofusin
   c. Transpulmonary contrast
   d. Omnipaque

4 What is the specific purpose of contrast in this case:
   a. Determine if ASD/PFO present
   b. Myocardial contrast imaging
   c. Determine if VSD present
   d. Rule out presence of thrombus

5 The following is also seen:
   a. Spontaneous echo contrast
   b. Mild–moderate MR
   c. Aortic dissection flap
   d. Dilated coronary sinus

Video Questions

CASE 20

VIDEOS 20.1, 20.2, 20.3, 20.4, 20.5, 20.6, 20.7, 20.8, 20.9, 20.10, 20.11

Questions

This 23-year-old woman presents with palpitations and exertional dyspnoea. She is found to have a loud, continuous murmur on auscultation. Her echo is shown.

Case Figure 20.1

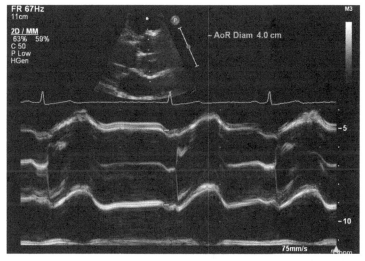

Case Figure 20.2

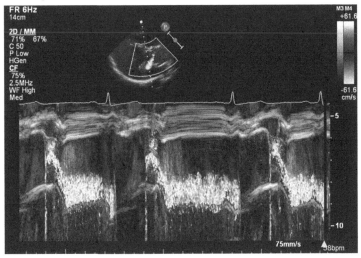

Case Figure 20.3

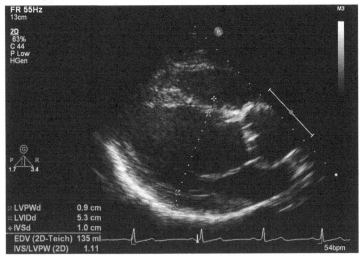

Case Figure 20.4

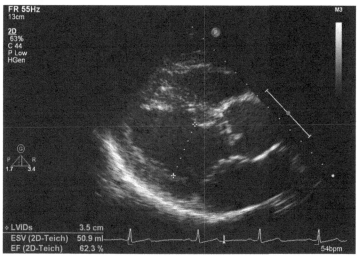

Case Figure 20.5

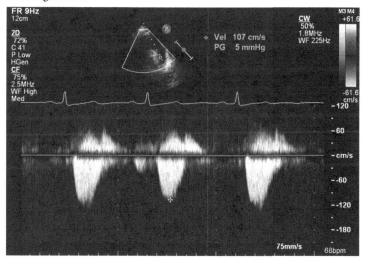

Case Figure 20.6

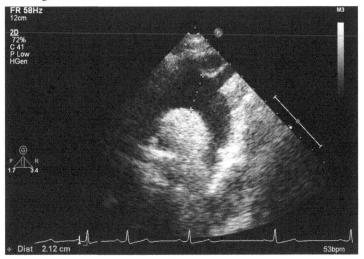

Select ONE option only for each of the questions below.

1 The following best describes the AR:
   a. Moderate, central
   b. Moderate, eccentric
   c. Severe, central
   d. Severe, eccentric

2 The following best describes the AV:
   a. Bicuspid with a very eccentric closure line
   b. Bicuspid with restricted leaflet opening
   c. Quadricuspid
   d. Bicuspid with a relatively central closure line

3 What other abnormality is demonstrated:
   a. VSD
   b. PDA
   c. ASD
   d. Coarctation of the aorta

4 The LV function is:
   a. Normal
   b. Mildly impaired
   c. Moderately impaired
   d. Severely impaired

5 The following statements are true regarding the findings in this study:

   a. Coarctation of the aorta should be sought as an association with bicuspid valves

   b. Monitoring of the aortic root size is important for follow-up even if asymptomatic

   c. Left ventricular dilatation is a complication of PDAs

   d. All of the above

Video Answers

Case 1
1 c.

An ASD occluder device is seen. Myxomas can be attached to the atrial septum but usually only by a stalk and are more mobile.

2 b.

The IVC collapses by around 50% on inspiration suggesting that RA pressure is approximately 10 mmHg. Hepatic veins distend as RA pressure increases.

3 d.

In most cases of ASDs, there is predominantly diastolic flow from left to right most commonly. Myxomas are far more common in the LA than RA. Ostium secundum defects can often be closed percutaneously. Thrombus crossing an ASD is well recognised although not very common.

4 e.

Both the RA and RV are dilated due to volume overload prior to the ASD closure. The LV function is normal and the estimated PA pressure is around 25–30 mmHg, which does not constitute pulmonary hypertension on echocardiography. Septal motion is normal in the parasternal views.

Case 2
1 c.

Myocardial contrast enhancement imaging has been performed to try and demonstrate vascularity. As the mass is right sided, embolisation into the pulmonary circulation would be more likely but not the systemic circulation.

2 b.

It appears localised around the RV.

3 e.

Each gradation on the M-mode callipers is 1 cm apart, so the LV cavity is clearly not dilated. None of the abnormalities listed are seen.

4 a.

The most likely diagnosis given the clinical scenario and the findings of a cardiac mass with a pericardial effusion is a tumour.

Case 3

1 a.

The transmitral flow E>A flow with normal deceleration slopes. In a 23-year-old woman with no symptoms, this is normal and not pseudonormalisation. A reversed E:A ratio would indicate impaired relaxation and steep deceleration slopes would indicate severe diastolic impairment.

2 a.

IVC collapse on inspiration is normal. There is no AR and LV function is normal. The subcostal colour flow does not show any evidence of an ASD.

3 e.

This is a dilated coronary sinus caused by the persistence of a left-sided SVC draining into the RA via the coronary sinus. All other options are far less likely given the clinical scenario.

4 d.

The AV is normal (tricuspid). As explained above, the dilated coronary sinus is due to a persistent left-sided SVC; injection of agitated saline into the left arm will opacify the coronary sinus only, confirming the suspicion. Injection of agitated saline into the right arm with valsalva will opacify the RV and RA (and may unmask a PFO if present) but will not help identify the abnormality in the LA.

Case 4

1 b.

The AR is mild on Doppler.

2 c.

The ascending aorta and arch are dilated but the descending aorta is normal. The TR is mild and the LVH is global and symmetrical.

3 d.

In Marfan's syndrome, dilatation of the aortic root or ascending aorta of >4.5 cm is an indication for surgery. The sinuses are classically flattened out in Ehlers–Danlos, so the normal shape of the aortic root is lost.

4 d.

The root is calcified, it is not prosthetic. The sinus measurements are normal. The apical 4-chamber view demonstrates systolic anterior motion of the anterior leaflet chordae of the MV.

Case 5

1 d.

There is no cavity obliteration. The LV is dilated at 6 cm end-diastole, with global, moderate impairment.

2 e.

All can potentially cause this appearance of moderate, global LV dysfunction.

3 a.

The AV is normal.

4 c.

The MV has thin and mobile leaflets with no significant abnormality.

Case 6

1 d.

This is Ebstein's anomaly.

2 a.

The colour Doppler shows aliasing suggesting a high velocity jet. It is an eccentric jet, directed against the 'ventricular' septum exhibiting the coanda effect, making the TR at least moderate.

3 c.

There is no evidence of MR.

4 e.
All are recognised associations.

Case 7
1 b.
The LVH is moderate and symmetrically affects the whole LV.

2 a.
The TAPSE suggests normal RV function.

3 e.
All are true.

4 a.
Ischaemic heart disease is the least likely cause as this would give thinned areas of myocardium with RWMA. All of the others are possible candidates.

Case 8
1 b.
This is the best fit answer.

2 e.
A gap is clearly seen within the centre section of the anterior MV leaflet in the parasternal long-axis and short-axis views.

3 b.
Mild TR is seen. The LA volume of up to 60 ml is normal. LV function is normal.

4 c.
The 3D image confirms the 2D findings that there is a cleft anterior MV leaflet.

Case 9
1 a.
This E:A reversal may be normal for the patient's age. More information would be required to decide on the presence of the other suggestions. E>A with short deceleration times would suggest severe diastolic dysfunction. Long pressure half times with high peak velocities would be in keeping with MS. Anything that

affects flow will affect the transmitral E and A velocities, such as anomalous pulmonary venous drainage and mitral regurgitation.

2 b.

The TR is mild–moderate by colour Doppler and by the intensity of the CW Doppler.

3 b.

It appears to show motion in association with the TV so this is the best fit answer. It is not associated with the atrial septum. It does not appear fluid filled, and its vascularity cannot be deduced from this study.

4 e.

The mass is the right heart and not the systemic side of the circulation so it is unlikely to have been responsible. The AV is not well seen and so no assessment of the number of cusps can be made, although its motion does not support it being bicuspid. The LV function is normal and there is no pericardial effusion.

Case 10

1 b.

The effusion is moderate (1.5 cm) with no evidence of haemodynamic compromise.

2 d.

The vegetation is attached to the posterior leaflet and the MR is directed anteriorly. This is best appreciated in the parasternal long-axis view.

3 c.

Acute, severe MR causes an increase in the EF as blood is ejected from the LV into the aorta and into the LA. European guidance suggests that an EF of <60% (by Simpson's method) suggests mild–moderate LV impairment in this situation.

4 d.

Embolic phenomena in the context of endocarditis should prompt consideration of surgery. Positive blood cultures are part of Duke's major criteria as is new valvular regurgitation.

Case 11

1 d.

Current BSE guidelines suggest wall thickness of ≥2 cm is in the severe category.

2 d.

There is no MR.

3 d.

All are true.

4 b.

The tissue Doppler imaging E:E' of the lateral wall is 21, which is markedly abnormal.

5 c.

Given the appearances of biventricular hypertrophy, valve thickening, decreased longitudinal contraction with preserved radial contraction and low QRS voltages on resting ECG, the most likely diagnosis is cardiac amyloidosis.

Case 12

1 d.

The LV function is hyperdynamic. Although calculated by M-mode, the EF is >65% and there is evidence of cavity obliteration in the 4-chamber view.

2 b.

The peak velocity and profile of the AV CW Doppler would suggest there is moderate AS.

3 a.

The RV function appears normal.

4 d.

PW Doppler shows maximum velocity of 1.8 m/s in the mid-ventricle, whereas CW Doppler shows peak velocity across the AV of 3.6 m/s with 2D imaging showing AV leaflet calcification and a profile more in keeping with AS rather than LVIT obstruction/cavity obliteration.

5 d.

It is the PW Doppler signal in the mid-ventricular level that shows the characteristic dagger-shaped profile of cavity obliteration.

Case 13

1 a.

Transmitral flow drops <25% with inspiration normally. Peak E wave velocity is 0.5 m/s, dropping to 0.4 m/s on inspiration. Peak A wave velocity drops from 0.65 m/s to 0.55 m/s. Both are <25%.

2 b.

This appearance is consistent with collapsed lung as a result of the large left pleural effusion.

3 a.

The RV contracts well in all views.

4 c.

Bilateral pleural effusions are seen with a small pericardial effusion.

Case 14

1 d.

The LV is globally, severely impaired visually. The EF is 35%.

2 c.

An adequate colour flow assessment across the MV is not seen and the CW Doppler profile shows interference from the aortic stenotic jet and so no reliable assessment of the severity of MR can be made from the study shown.

3 d.

The LVH is symmetrical and moderate in severity.

4 d.

The effusion is small, non-compromising and global. This is best appreciated on the subcostal view.

5 d.

As the LV function is impaired, the AV area, as measured by the continuity equation, is the best measure of severity.

Case 15

1 d.

All are seen.

2 d.

Again, all are shown in this case.

3 b.

The LV is dilated, and the MR is severe and eccentric. Calculation of the MR regurgitant fraction requires the PISA measurement, aliasing velocity and the peak velocity of the MR regurgitant jet, all of which can be assessed from the data provided, although this may not always be accurate when regurgitant jets are eccentric. The colour M-mode of the AR jet shows around 20–30% LVOT width.

4 b.

As the jet is eccentric, vena contracta is the most accurate measure of severity.

5 b.

P2 prolapse is clearly seen in the apical long-axis views.

Case 16

1 c.

The LV is clearly dilated at end-diastole and is severely impaired.

2 d.

This cannot be assessed on the TR velocity alone as the RA pressure is likely to be raised given the RV impairment. Hence, IVC assessment is required.

3 d.

The most likely diagnosis is non-ischaemic dilated cardiomyopathy

4 a.

He does not have significant coronary artery disease. He fits NICE criteria for consideration of CRT.

5 b.

The most likely aetiology with an LVEDD of 6.8 cm and normal coronary arteries, is functional MR secondary to annular dilatation.

Case 17

1 c.

The pressure half time gives the best assessment of severity from the images provided.

2 d.

The AR is severe because the pressure half time is <250 ms

3 a.

The LV function is normal to slightly hyperdynamic as a result of the volume overload to the LV.

4 b.

There is a mobile mass attached to it. It is not artefact and is not any of the normal variants e.g. nodules of Arantius or Lambl's excrescences.

5 b.

It is likely that this man developed AV endocarditis following his dental surgery. This has resulted in severe AR that is now the cause of his presenting symptoms.

Case 18

1 c.

The pulmonary artery is seen exiting the morphological LV and bifurcating into the left and right main branches.

2 a.

The TV is the most apically positioned of the two atrioventricular valves. It is draining the LA (with pulmonary veins seen draining into it) into the systemic ventricle, which in this case is the morphological RV (moderator band is seen in it).

3 a.

There is no MR; it is TR that is seen.

4 d.

All are seen.

5 e.

This is congenitally corrected transposition of the great arteries. The patient was born with atrioventricular dissociation (i.e. LA drains into morphological RV, and RA drains into morphological LV) and ventriculo-arterial dissociation (i.e. morphological LV exits into PA, and morphological RV exits into aorta) and now presents with symptoms of systemic ventricular failure.

Case 19
1 c.

The most likely explanation is the presence of the RV pacing lead even though this is not seen. The ECG shows a paced rhythm. There is mild–moderate TR into a non-dilated RA.

2 d.

This is the best fit answer.

3 c.

Contrast is seen first in filling the RV and subsequently filling the LV; this identifies it as transpulmonary contrast.

4 d.

This is to exclude the presence of thrombus in the LV apex prior to cannulation of the apex with an LVAD.

5 b.

Mild–moderate MR is also seen, which should regress following implantation of the LVAD.

Case 20
1 b.

The jet is clearly eccentric, and colour M-mode on the LVOT shows between 20–60% LVOT width, with no flow reversal seen in the aortic arch. This would be in keeping with moderate AR.

2 d.

The AV is bicuspid but has a fairly central closure line, which is unusual.

3 b.

The suprasternal view demonstrates a communication between the PA and the descending aorta. This is a PDA and explains her continuous murmur. The PDA is also seen in the parasternal short axis.

4 a.

The LV function is normal.

5 d.

All are true.

Index

Chapters 1 to 8 are referenced in the form of chapter and question number(s) (e.g. 2.9 or 3.9–11). Chapter 9 is referenced in the form of chapter, then case, followed by question number (e.g. 9c3.1).

Successful Accreditation in Echocardiography: A Self-Assessment Guide,
First Edition. Sanjay M. Banypersad and Keith Pearce.
© 2012 John Wiley & Sons, Ltd. Published 2012 by John Wiley & Sons, Ltd.

Printed in the United States
By Bookmasters